INTERMITTENT FASTING BASICS

FOR WOMEN

INCLUDES EASY-TO-FOLLOW MEAL PLANS

The Complete Guide to Safe and Effective Weight Loss with Intermittent Fasting

FASTING GUIDELINES

MEAL PLANNING

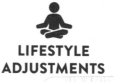

LIFESTYLE ADJUSTMENTS

LINDSAY BOYERS, CHNC

Adams Media
New York London Toronto Sydney New Delhi

T0001305

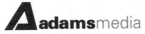

Adams Media
An Imprint of Simon & Schuster, Inc.
57 Littlefield Street
Avon, Massachusetts 02322

Copyright © 2021 by Simon & Schuster, Inc.

First Adams Media trade paperback edition April 2021

ADAMS MEDIA and colophon are trademarks of Simon & Schuster.

For information about special discounts for bulk purchases, please contact Simon & Schuster Special Sales at 1-866-506-1949 or business@simonandschuster.com.

The Simon & Schuster Speakers Bureau can bring authors to your live event. For more information or to book an event contact the Simon & Schuster Speakers Bureau at 1-866-248-3049 or visit our website at www.simonspeakers.com.

Interior images © Getty Images

Manufactured in the United States of America

1 2021

Library of Congress Cataloging-in-Publication Data has been applied for.

ISBN 978-1-5072-1570-8
ISBN 978-1-5072-1571-5 (ebook)

Contents

Chapter 2: Why Women Are More Sensitive to Fasting 39

Chapter 3: Getting a Handle on Stress and Hormones......................75

Chapter 4: Best Fasting Approaches for Women 105

Chapter 7: Meal Plans..189

Introduction

You may have heard about the health benefits of fasting. Not only does it help you shed stubborn pounds; it also increases energy, reduces inflammation, and may even reduce your risk of heart disease (the leading cause of death in women in the United States). But where do you begin?

With the basics. *Intermittent Fasting Basics for Women* teaches you everything you need to know about fasting as a woman, in a quick, easy-to-understand way. Not sure how exactly intermittent fasting works? You'll learn about the mechanisms of autophagy, as well as the truth behind common misunderstandings about starvation mode, cutting carbohydrates, and more. Wondering about the differences between fasting for men versus for women? You'll uncover the unique factors that impact your body and how it reacts to fasting, from your hormones to the effects of stress—and why women are especially susceptible to these effects.

Unsure of which fasting approach is right for you? This book explores each of the fasting schedules recommended for women, as well as various meal plans you may work your fasting routine into, including keto and vegan plans. Plus, each meal plan includes easy recipes to help you reap the full benefits *and* stick to your fasting schedule.

Whether you're brand-new to intermittent fasting, or you've tried it before but haven't had much success, this book is here to help you apply this lifestyle to your unique needs—easily and effectively.

1

Intermittent Fasting Basics

You may be hearing a lot about intermittent fasting recently, but it's not new. In fact, one of the oldest known scientific studies on intermittent fasting dates back seventy-five years! And the concept as a whole goes back even further to the days of hunting and gathering—even if your ancestors weren't doing it on purpose. Intermittent fasting has stood the test of time because it isn't just another diet. It's a powerful eating strategy that has profound effects when done correctly. While intermittent fasting can certainly help you lose weight, its health benefits go way beyond that. It can also increase your energy, improve your concentration, reduce puffiness and inflammation, and help protect you—and your brain—from various chronic diseases.

There's some confusion surrounding intermittent fasting, though. Some people think it's just a fancy way of restricting calories, but it's so much more than that. In this chapter, you'll learn the basics of intermittent fasting and why it's so powerful. You'll also discover the difference between intermittent fasting and calorie restriction and why you should kick low-calorie diets to the curb forever.

What Is Intermittent Fasting?

Intermittent fasting is a nonspecific term for cycling between periods of fasting and eating. There are several types of intermittent fasting, but they all share one major commonality: Instead of focusing primarily on *what* you eat, you pay more attention to *when* you eat (although that doesn't mean the quality of your diet isn't also important).

According to Dr. Mark Mattson, a researcher on intermittent fasting and professor of neuroscience at Johns Hopkins University, the human body is designed to go without food for several hours to several days, but after the Industrial Revolution, food became accessible all the time. As a result, the human diet changed significantly, and biology hasn't caught up yet. People are eating more food more often, and these extra calories (coupled with sedentary lifestyles) have led to chronic health issues like obesity, type 2 diabetes, and heart disease, which is the leading cause of death for women in the United States.

When you go for set periods of time without food, it allows your body to properly focus on digestion and deplete your energy—or glucose—stores so that your metabolism is forced to start burning your own body fat. Mattson defines this process as "metabolic switching." Keep in mind that body fat is just excessive food energy that's been stored; if you continue to eat more than you need, that excess energy has to find somewhere to go, and body fat will continue to increase. On the other hand, when you fast, your body turns to its own fat for an energy source.

The Fed State

The fed state, also called the absorptive stage, occurs right after you eat a meal or snack. As soon as you eat, your body starts to work on breaking down the food and absorbing the nutrients from it. Components of this digested material enter your blood, causing blood glucose levels to rise. The rise of glucose then triggers the beta cells in your pancreas to release insulin, which binds to receptors in your cells, stimulating them to open and let glucose in. Once glucose is inside your cells, three things happen:

1. It's used as a direct source of energy by your cells.
2. It's converted to glycogen and stored in your liver and muscles for later use.
3. It's converted `into triglycerides and stored in your body as fat.

You're technically in a fed state until all of the digested material travels out of the gastrointestinal tract. When you're in a fed state:

- Insulin is high.
- Glucose is high.
- You're using glucose as energy.
- You're storing fat.

Depending on what you eat, a fed state typically lasts about four hours after you eat, so if you never let more than at least four hours pass between meals or snacks, your body will consistently remain in a fed state.

The Fasted State

The fasted state, also called the postabsorptive phase, occurs after your food has been fully digested, absorbed, and stored. All of the digested materials have moved out of the gastrointestinal tract, glucose in your bloodstream has leveled off, and your body is now turning toward stored glycogen for energy.

When glucose levels in the blood drop, insulin levels also drop. In order to keep glucose levels between 70 and 99 milligrams per deciliter (the normal range for adults), the alpha cells in your pancreas release glucagon—a hormone that travels to the liver and helps convert glycogen back into glucose. The glucose then travels to your cells and provides energy to your brain and tissues.

When you're in a fasted state:

- Insulin is low.
- Glucose is low.
- Your body starts breaking down fat for energy.
- You're burning fat.

Because the fed state lasts for four hours, and you typically don't enter the fasted state until after four hours after your last meal, it's rare for your body to enter this fat-burning state—unless you time your food intake. This is one of the reasons why many women lose weight and body fat when they start intermittent fasting, even if they don't change anything else they're doing. Fasting forces your body into that fat-burning state that you rarely reach during a normal eating schedule.

When Your Body Starts Burning Fat

Your liver can store about 100–120 grams of glycogen, while your muscles can hold onto about 400–500 grams. How long this glycogen lasts depends on how much movement you're doing—it will last longer when you're just sitting on the couch watching *Netflix* than if you're running a marathon—but in general, you'll get about an hour and a half to two hours of energy out of your stored glycogen before it's depleted.

Most people never get this far, though. If you're following advice to eat every few hours to avoid "starvation mode" (discussed later in this chapter), you're constantly refilling your glycogen stores, so you're also constantly using glycogen for energy. On the other hand, when you fast, you allow your glucose and glycogen to burn up to the point that your body has to look somewhere else for the energy it needs and it turns to your own body fat.

When glucose and glycogen levels diminish, your body starts to break down the fats in your body into glycerol and fatty acids through a process called lipolysis. Glycerol is taken to your liver where it undergoes a process called gluconeogenesis. During gluconeogenesis, glycerol is converted into glucose and glycogen so that it can help replenish your liver glycogen stores. This process is essential because your brain and central nervous system rely on sugar for energy. Some of the free fatty acids are transported to your muscle tissues where they're used as energy, and others go to your liver where they're broken down and converted into ketones through a process called beta-oxidation.

What Are Ketones?

Ketones have more recently earned their time in the spotlight due to the increasing popularity of the ketogenic, or keto, diet, but humans have been relying on ketones as a source of energy for hundreds of years.

In simple terms, ketones, also called ketone bodies, are chemicals made by your liver when there's not enough glucose in your body to supply the energy you need. These ketones, which are made from fatty acids, provide an alternative source of fuel, or energy, for your body so you can carry out the normal physiological functions that keep you alive.

Ketones can help improve cognitive function and mental performance because they can easily cross the blood-brain barrier and supply a quick-acting source of energy to your brain. Ketones also provide a steady supply of physical energy for your body. That's why many people experience increased energy when following a ketogenic diet or incorporating intermittent fasting.

There are three types of ketones:

- Acetoacetate (AcAc)
- Beta-hydroxybutyrate (BHB)
- Acetone

Your liver produces ketones all of the time, but the concentration of ketones in your blood relies heavily on your carbohydrate and protein intake and how often you eat. While high levels of ketones can be dangerous for someone with type 1 diabetes, someone with a properly functioning metabolism can handle them with no problem. Any extra ketones that your body doesn't use as energy will be excreted when you breathe or pee.

Fasting and Ketosis

It typically takes about twelve hours of fasting to reach the fat-burning state of ketosis, and things continue to ramp up around hours sixteen to twenty-four. That's why many people recommend fasting for sixteen hours. However, while this time frame seems to work really well for men, women typically do better with shorter fasts, around twelve to fourteen hours.

While you'll start to burn fat after around twelve hours, you don't actually enter into full nutritional ketosis. That process takes two to four days on average, assuming you're eating fewer than 50 grams of carbohydrates per day. While the body does create some ketones during fasting, it's usually not enough to say you're in ketosis.

According to a March 2017 report in *Sports Medicine*, ketone body concentrations remain relatively low (in the range of about 0.1–0.5 mmol/l) after an overnight fast. To put that into perspective, researchers Stephen Phinney and Jeff Volek, two widely recognized experts on fasting, recommend blood ketone levels of 1.5–3.0 mmol/l to achieve nutritional ketosis and gain the best weight-loss effects. This is why many women choose to combine intermittent fasting with a ketogenic diet—a high-fat dietary plan that limits carbohydrate intake to no more than 50 grams per day.

Don't You Need Carbohydrates to Survive?

You may have reservations about following a ketogenic diet. After all, you need carbohydrates to survive, right? Not exactly. You need *glucose* to survive. While carbohydrates are an easy source of glucose for your body, you don't have to eat carbs to get glucose. If you haven't figured it out yet, your body is incredible, and in the absence of carbohydrates, it will use other sources to make the glucose it needs.

To be clear, not all of your cells need glucose, but certain important organs and structures, like your liver and your red blood cells, can't function efficiently without a sugar source. Your brain can't run directly on fatty acids, but it can use ketones effectively.

When your body breaks down fat, it creates glycerol that gets converted into glucose through gluconeogenesis. But this is not the only source of glucose when you're fasting or restricting carbohydrates. Your body can also make glucose from the amino acids in protein or from lactate, a waste product produced by your muscles during exercise and movement.

Gluconeogenesis and ketogenesis have a synergistic relationship. When you fast—or you restrict carbohydrates to mimic fasting—it starts the process of ketogenesis, which creates the ketones that supply energy to your muscles, brain, heart, kidneys, and many other cells. At the same time, fasting or carbohydrate restriction prompts gluconeogenesis, which creates the glucose that provides energy to your red blood cells and liver and helps keep your blood sugar levels within normal, healthy ranges.

What about Starvation Mode?

If you're new to the idea of skipping meals, your first thought may be "But what about starvation mode?" It's a common concern, but the truth is that starvation mode is a fallacy—at least, in the way it's typically presented. Many people say that you will enter starvation mode if you skip a meal or don't eat often enough. That's where the idea of eating several small meals, instead of three large ones, came from. In fact, when someone who's dieting reaches a weight-loss plateau, oftentimes the advice is that they're not eating enough and simply need to eat more often to prevent the body from entering starvation mode. But it doesn't work quite like that.

Starvation mode, the technical name for adaptive thermogenesis, is your body's physiological response to a severe calorie deficit, not skipping a few meals here and there. When you severely restrict calories, your body interprets that as a threat to survival. As a result, your central nervous system and your hormones work together to slow down your metabolism and conserve energy so that it's harder to lose body fat.

If you remain in this calorie-restricted state for too long, it can cause hormonal imbalances and increased difficulty maintaining a healthy weight. At this point, it now becomes classified as metabolic damage—a physiological condition that can cause even more severe hormonal imbalances (especially with the hunger hormones) and muscle loss.

Because intermittent fasting isn't a severe restriction of calories, it doesn't trigger adaptive thermogenesis. It actually does the opposite. When you focus on meal timing, rather than severe calorie restriction, it helps balance hormones, preserve lean muscle mass, and improve your metabolism. When done right, intermittent fasting can even reverse metabolic damage and metabolic syndrome.

Intermittent Fasting versus Calorie Restriction

Intermittent fasting may seem like just a fancy name for calorie restriction, but the two approaches to eating aren't the same. Calorie restriction involves lowering your daily calorie intake in an effort to lose weight. Most calorie-restricted diets don't have set guidelines on when you can eat, but there are usually certain foods that are off-limits.

With intermittent fasting, you restrict eating to predetermined windows of time. In other words, you eat only during certain time periods. Because you have less time to eat during the day, intermittent fasting may naturally lead to calorie restriction, but eating fewer calories isn't the main goal.

If weight loss is your goal, both eating methods will help you get there, but intermittent fasting has several advantages over daily calorie restriction. In a review published in *Obesity Reviews* in 2011, researchers looked over all of the studies on intermittent fasting and calorie restriction and found that while both methods prompt a similar amount of weight loss, people tend to retain more lean muscle mass with intermittent fasting. In other words, intermittent fasting helps improve your body composition, or lessen your body fat percentage, rather than just lowering the number on the scale.

Other studies show that intermittent fasting is more effective at balancing the hunger hormones, ghrelin and leptin, so these kinds of diets are easier to maintain for the long haul. On the other hand, many women who rely on calorie restriction as a method of weight loss end up regaining the weight once they go back to eating a normal amount of calories.

The Downsides of Calorie Restriction

While calorie restriction is an effective way to lose weight initially, maintaining that weight loss is another story. Studies show that sustained calorie deficits—or restricting your calorie intake for a long period of time—can increase the strength and frequency of food cravings in women and increase the desire to use food as a reward.

Reducing calorie intake triggers hormonal changes that increase your appetite, decrease your metabolic rate, and make you want to eat high-calorie foods. Here are the main hormones that are negatively affected by calorie restriction:

- Leptin
- Peptide YY
- Cholecystokinin
- Insulin
- Ghrelin
- Gastric inhibitory polypeptide
- Pancreatic polypeptide

What's even more unsettling is that these negative hormonal changes can persist for over a year even after you stop dieting, according to research published in *Perspectives on Psychological Science* in 2017.

That's why when you focus only on restricting calories, you feel hungry all the time and have a hard time focusing on anything but food. Your hormones are so out of whack that they're constantly telling your body you need to eat, even if you just had a meal. Because your metabolism is also slowing down, you'll have to continue dropping your daily calorie intake to continue seeing results. One- to two-thirds of people who restrict calories as a means to weight loss not only gain all the weight back, but they also regain even more weight than they lost in the first place!

Intermittent Fasting Helps Control Your Hunger

It makes sense to think that fasting would lead to increased hunger, but once your body adapts, the opposite happens. It's true that in the beginning stages, when you're getting used to the idea of skipping meals, you may feel hungry more often, but usually this is more of a psychological response. When you're used to eating whenever you want and you suddenly tell your body it can't have food after a certain time, it rebels, wanting it more. If you stick with your schedule, you will naturally adjust after a week or two.

This is because intermittent fasting helps balance the two main hormones involved in hunger: ghrelin and leptin. Ghrelin is nicknamed the "hunger hormone" because when levels go up, you feel hungry. It is produced in your stomach and sends signals to your brain that glucose levels are low, so you need to eat. Leptin is called the "satiation hormone." It does the opposite of ghrelin. When leptin levels go up, you feel satisfied and signals are sent to your brain saying that you're full and it's time to stop eating. Leptin is produced by your adipose, or fat, tissue.

Unlike the way calorie restriction, which negatively affects ghrelin and leptin, leaves you feeling hungry all the time, and can often lead to obsession with food, intermittent fasting can lower ghrelin while simultaneously increasing leptin, allowing you to feel fully satisfied. This helps you stop eating naturally, instead of forcing restrictions on you based solely on calorie count.

Feeling satisfied and keeping hunger at bay is a benefit in itself, but this is especially beneficial if you're trying to lose weight. Leptin resistance, a condition in which the body doesn't respond appropriately to leptin, is one of the leading underlying mechanisms in weight and fat gain in women. Leptin resistance is also closely tied to insulin resistance—and intermittent fasting has been shown to improve both.

What Is Leptin Resistance?

Many experts believe that leptin resistance, a condition in which your body doesn't respond appropriately to the hormone leptin, is the underlying driver of fat gain and obesity. To understand why this happens, you have to know how leptin is made and what it does.

Leptin is made in your fat, or adipose, tissue. Ordinarily, fat cells release leptin, which travels to the hypothalamus in your brain. The brain senses that leptin and sends out signals that you're full and can stop eating. This feedback system is intended to help keep you at a healthy weight and prevent you from gaining too many fat cells.

However, there are many women who are leptin resistant and don't respond well to leptin. For someone who's leptin resistant, this feedback system looks different: The fat cells release leptin, and the leptin travels through your bloodstream, but the hypothalamus doesn't sense it. As a result, your fat cells continue to produce more leptin. Leptin levels in the blood stay high, but your brain never actually gets the signal that you're full. This leptin overload eventually causes your leptin response to shut down completely, and, as a result, it becomes increasingly difficult to control your appetite. You always feel hungry and have to force yourself to stop eating, instead of just naturally feeling full. Or, you just continue to eat, accumulating more fat cells, which continue to produce leptin and perpetuate the broken cycle.

This is the very system that makes overweight or obese women feel like they are starving. It's not about laziness or lack of willpower. Your body literally cannot read the signals that you're full.

How Fasting Helps Improve Leptin Resistance

In some cases, leptin resistance can be a sign of a more serious underlying issue, but the majority of time, it develops as a result of years of poor diet and lifestyle choices.

Some things that can cause leptin resistance are:

- Lack of sleep
- Lots of stress
- High-fat, high-carbohydrate diets
- Chronic inflammation
- High levels of insulin/insulin resistance

If you really want to get a handle on your health and be able to effortlessly maintain a healthy weight while also feeling completely satisfied, you have to make sure your body is responding to and utilizing leptin correctly. And intermittent fasting is a great way to do that.

When you fast, it can help balance your blood sugar and insulin levels, and, according to Dr. Jason Fung, an expert on intermittent fasting, the key to improving leptin resistance is lowering insulin levels. In addition to fasting, you can also lower your insulin levels by:

- Eating less sugar and refined grains
- Eating moderate protein and lots of high-quality fats
- Eating whole, unprocessed foods

Intermittent fasting can also help reduce body fat. Since leptin is created in your fat tissue, reducing the amount of body fat you have will naturally reduce leptin levels so that you can turn off the overload on your system and start appropriately responding to leptin again.

Trimming Your Waistline

Intermittent fasting can prompt weight loss, trim your waistline, and improve metabolism even without restricting calories. In one review published in *Canadian Family Physician* in 2020, researchers compared results of twenty-seven different intermittent fasting trials. They found that participants lost weight in every single study, with an average total weight loss of 0.8–13 percent of starting body weight in a period of two to twenty-six weeks.

The studies incorporated different types of fasting and different types of dietary plans, from Mediterranean-style diets to moderate fat, low-carb diets to high-protein diets. Some of the studies even followed the American Heart Association's recommendations of 55 percent carbohydrates, 25 percent protein, and 20 percent fat. No matter what the specific details of their diet were, all of the participants lost weight. The only common denominator was that all had incorporated fasting.

In another study published in *Translational Research* in 2014, fasting helped participants lose 4–7 percent of their total waist circumference, which means they specifically lost the dangerous type of fat called visceral fat. Visceral fat, often described as biologically active fat, is stored inside the abdominal cavity close to several major organs, including the liver, stomach, pancreas, and intestines. Having a lot of visceral fat increases your risk of heart disease, diabetes, stroke, depression, cancer, and arthritis. Because visceral fat is biologically active, it can also negatively affect your hormones.

In a study published in the *Journal of Diabetes & Metabolic Disorders* in 2013, women were instructed to eat their usual diet but incorporate intermittent fasting every other day. Without any other changes, on average, the women lost about 13 pounds and decreased their waist circumference by 5 centimeters after just two months.

Improving Your Metabolic Health

When you hear the word *metabolism*, you may immediately associate it with your weight and how many calories you burn, but that's only a small part of how your metabolism intersects with your overall health.

Metabolic health is defined as having healthy blood sugar, triglycerides, HDL cholesterol, blood pressure, and waist circumference without taking any medications. According to a 2019 study from the University of North Carolina at Chapel Hill's Gillings School of Global Public Health, only about 12 percent of Americans have good metabolic health.

Not only does poor metabolic health increase your risk of complications from viral and bacterial infections; it also makes it more likely that you'll develop heart disease (or have a stroke), diabetes, or cancer. Your diet and eating habits play a huge role in your metabolic health, but even if your weight is considered normal, that doesn't necessarily mean you're metabolically healthy. You could still have underlying issues that may make you more susceptible to chronic disease.

Fasting is one way to start improving things. Studies show that intermittent fasting can improve your metabolic health, which reduces your risk of chronic diseases and obesity, increases your longevity, and makes you more resilient and resistant to the negative effects of stress. Fasting also improves metabolic flexibility. When you're metabolically flexible, your body can use whatever source of energy you give it. This is beneficial because it means you can burn carbs when you eat carbs or burn fat when you eat fat, instead of either of them prompting more significant weight gain than the other.

If you get "hangry" or irritable when you haven't eaten for a few hours, there's a good chance you're metabolically inflexible. Intermittent fasting is a great way to fix that.

You Burn More Calories Too

There's pervasive advice that the way to optimize your calorie burn is to eat small amounts of food more often to avoid entering *starvation mode*, which is a term used to describe a metabolic slowdown (and resulting decrease in calorie burn) due to skipping meals or restricting calories. While the recommendation to graze all day is well intentioned, it's entirely misguided. The only way your body would enter into starvation mode is if you go several days or weeks without eating, you're extremely malnourished, and you've burned through all of your body fat.

That type of metabolic slowdown doesn't happen in a matter of hours. If it did, the human species wouldn't have survived prior to the Industrial Revolution when food scarcity was common.

Thankfully, the human body is much smarter and more advanced than this. Research shows that intermittent fasting doesn't trigger starvation mode and hinder your ability to burn calories and fat. It actually has the opposite effect on your metabolic rate. According to two studies—one in the *American Journal of Physiology* and another in *The American Journal of Clinical Nutrition*—your basal metabolic rate (BMR), or the number of calories you burn while at rest, increases significantly after periods of short-term fasting.

When you enter a fasted state, your body increases the production of norepinephrine, a stress hormone and neurotransmitter that stimulates your metabolism and triggers your body to break down excess fat. Intermittent fasting also increases production of human growth hormone (HGH), which breaks down fat and increases lean muscle mass—a combination that helps you burn more calories at rest.

Fat As an Energy Source

Increased energy is one of the first benefits many women report when first implementing intermittent fasting. One reason for this is that intermittent fasting allows food to fully digest and leave the digestive tract. When you're in that fasted state, you naturally feel lighter and less sluggish. No more going to bed full and bloated and waking up with stomach cramps and pain.

Another reason that fasting can benefit your energy levels is that fat is an extremely efficient energy source. Not only does your body use fat quickly and easily, but fat also provides 9 calories per gram compared to the 4 calories per gram provided by protein and carbohydrates.

Your body can also store an unlimited supply of fat. Unlike glucose and glycogen, which run out after several hours, there's no limit to how much fat your body can store. Of course, that doesn't mean you want to go overboard and eat more than you need, but it's nice to know that you can train your body to run off of this extremely efficient energy source.

Fasting Balances Blood Sugar and Insulin Levels

Unbalanced blood sugar and insulin are the underlying cause of many of today's chronic health issues, like metabolic syndrome, type 2 diabetes, insulin resistance, and obesity. It's currently estimated that 15 million American women—or around 11 percent—have type 2 diabetes, while around 40–45 percent are obese and at risk of developing chronic health conditions, if they don't have one or more already.

Even if you don't have a chronic disease, low blood sugar—or poor blood sugar regulation—can cause:

- Irritability
- Anxiety
- Confusion
- Dizziness
- Fatigue
- Headache
- Shakiness
- Blurred vision
- Dry mouth
- Increased perspiration

When you eat all the time, your blood sugar and insulin levels are constantly rising and dropping throughout the day, but the degree to which they rise and drop depends on what you're eating. Refined carbohydrates like sugar and white bread cause more dramatic spikes and dips, while natural complex carbohydrates like sweet potatoes and black beans will have more moderate effects. If you're constantly spiking your blood sugar and insulin levels throughout the day, it can lead to chronically high blood sugar levels and, eventually, insulin resistance.

On the other hand, when you make intermittent fasting a regular part of your routine, you teach your body to burn fat for energy instead of relying on glucose. This not only lowers blood sugar and insulin levels; it also improves overall insulin sensitivity.

Balanced blood sugar levels are also associated with:

- Improved fasting blood glucose (blood sugar levels after going twelve hours without food)
- Improved postprandial blood glucose (blood sugar levels right after eating a meal)
- Reduced glucose variability (dramatic spikes and dips in blood sugar levels)

All of this translates to weight loss, increased energy, improved mood, and a lower chance of developing type 2 diabetes and all of the complications that can come with it.

The Problem with Chronic Inflammation

There are two types of inflammation: acute and chronic. Acute inflammation is a normal immune response that occurs in response to an immediate threat. When you get sick or injured, inflammation turns on to help you heal; when the threat is gone, the inflammation goes away. Chronic inflammation is another beast entirely.

Your body experiences chronic inflammation in response to what it perceives as a threat, except this threat is long-lasting and not always obvious. Chronic inflammation can develop due to an undiagnosed food sensitivity or in response to prolonged, unmanaged stress. It can occur as a result of eating lots of sugar or not getting enough sleep. Chronic inflammation can last months to years, and, if left untreated, it can cause scarring and thickening in the connective tissue that can eventually lead to tissue death.

Researchers have linked chronic inflammation to:

- Autoimmune diseases
- Obesity
- Ulcerative colitis and Crohn's disease
- Heart disease
- Asthma
- Alzheimer's disease
- Cancer
- Polycystic ovary syndrome (PCOS)

Even if chronic inflammation hasn't developed into a diagnosable disease or condition, it can cause lingering symptoms that interfere with your quality of life.

Some of these symptoms include:

- Generalized dull, aching pain that affects the muscles and joints
- Stiffness and swelling
- Fatigue
- Insomnia and/or poor-quality sleep (e.g., waking up tired in the morning)
- Depression
- Anxiety
- Mood swings
- Abdominal pain
- Gas and bloating
- Constipation or diarrhea
- Acid reflux

Research shows that intermittent fasting can help reduce chronic inflammation by blocking inflammasomes and pro-inflammatory substances called leukotrienes.

Reducing Chronic Inflammation

Intermittent fasting helps reduce chronic inflammation in two major ways. Chronic inflammation is triggered, in part, by a substance called NLRP3, which is categorized as an inflammasome. Inflammasomes like NLRP3 are connected to the development of metabolic diseases, like diabetes and nonalcoholic fatty liver disease, and neurodegenerative diseases, like dementia, Parkinson's disease, and Huntington's disease. When you fast, your body produces a ketone called beta-hydroxybutyrate (BHB). BHB acts directly on NLRP3, shutting off the inflammatory response and helping reduce chronic inflammation and its negative effects.

Intermittent fasting also reduces the creation and release of leukotrienes, pro-inflammatory substances that are made by your white blood cells. Small amounts of leukotrienes are helpful for responding to acute inflammation and fighting off immediate threats, but excess production can contribute to chronic inflammation and the development of inflammatory and allergic diseases, like asthma and rheumatoid arthritis, which affects women three times more often than men. Women also tend to get rheumatoid arthritis earlier in life and usually have more severe symptoms.

When you eliminate chronic inflammation, you'll probably notice that puffiness in your face, hands, and feet goes away. You may feel and look slimmer, and your skin may look tighter and more vibrant. Chronic aches and pains that have just become a normal part of your day may start to diminish or even go away completely. It's also likely that you'll fall asleep faster, stay in a deeper sleep longer, and wake up feeling refreshed and ready to start your day, instead of dragging yourself out of bed when your alarm goes off.

Keeping Your Heart Healthy

Heart disease is the leading cause of death in women, killing more than a quarter of a million women every year in the US alone and affecting millions more. The Centers for Disease Control and Prevention estimates that 80 percent of deaths that occur as a result of coronary artery disease can be attributed to preventable factors like poor diet, high cholesterol and high blood pressure, obesity, excess alcohol consumption, and lack of exercise.

In addition to measuring weight loss in women, a study in the *Journal of Diabetes & Metabolic Disorders* measured markers for heart disease, like blood pressure, cholesterol levels, triglycerides, and body fat percentage. Here's what happened after an eight-week period of alternate-day fasting, but no other changes in diet or lifestyle:

- Systolic blood pressure went down by about 10 mm Hg.
- Diastolic blood pressure went down by about 8 mm Hg.
- Total cholesterol went down by 13 mg/dl.
- LDL cholesterol went down by 18 mg/dl.
- HDL cholesterol went up by 8 mg/dl.
- Triglycerides went down 17 mg/dl.
- Body fat percentage went down by 3 percent.

Other studies have shown 25 percent reductions in LDL cholesterol, often called "bad cholesterol," and 32 percent reductions in triglyceride levels in participants who incorporated fasting into their lifestyle. But what's even more important is that fasting specifically targets small, dense LDL particles, the ones that can get in your arterial walls and lead to atherosclerosis and heart disease.

Improving Your Brain Health

Brain fog and fatigue are two of the most common complaints of women today. And these symptoms can worsen as you reach perimenopause and menopause. In fact, 60 percent of women in the US report cognitive issues like impaired thinking and short-term memory loss when hormones start to change. But even though these symptoms are common, that doesn't mean they're normal.

Unstable hormones, high blood sugar, insulin resistance, excessive sugar intake, stress, and excess weight all can contribute to impaired brain function. Because intermittent fasting can help correct these conditions, it can also lead to significant improvements in cognitive symptoms. In addition, intermittent fasting increases the rate of neurogenesis, or the creation of new brain cells and nerve tissues in your brain, according to Dr. Mark Mattson, PhD, a professor of neuroscience at Johns Hopkins University. Increased neurogenesis has been connected to better memory and focus, improved mood, and boosts in overall brain function.

Intermittent fasting also increases the production of brain-derived neurotrophic factor (BDNF), a protein that increases the brain's production of new neurons and helps strengthen the connections between the neurons that are already there, while also increasing human growth hormone (HGH), which helps the body create new brain cells, protects the brain from damage, and improves cognition. High levels of BDNF also help improve mood, increase motivation, and decrease rates of depression.

Protecting You from Cancer

After heart disease, cancer is the second leading cause of death in US women. While you may feel like you're just a victim of your genes, the American Cancer Society estimates that at least 42 percent of cancer cases and 45 percent of cancer deaths could be prevented by changing your lifestyle.

Intermittent fasting helps improve insulin sensitivity, which makes it harder for cancer cells to grow and develop. It can also reduce obesity and type 2 diabetes, two conditions that are linked to higher rates of cancer and lower survival rates. But intermittent fasting may also help directly inhibit cancer.

Animal studies show that intermittent fasting can reduce tumor growth, decrease the cancer's ability to spread, and improve survival rates. While no official claims can be made for humans, this research is certainly promising.

Intermittent fasting and fasting-mimicking diets are also shown to reduce the cancer cells' ability to adapt and survive, which can improve the outcome of current cancer therapies. Remarkably, intermittent fasting can promote regeneration of new cells in normal tissues and increase normal cells' resistance to chemotherapy, with no effect on cancer cells. In other words, intermittent fasting can help normal cells survive chemotherapy treatments while cancer cells die, a combination that could improve chemotherapy outcomes, reduce side effects, and even prevent treatment-associated death.

Some animal studies show that fasting, combined with high-dose vitamin C, can help fight tumors in hard-to-treat mutated cancers. Of course, if you've been diagnosed with cancer, it's important to follow your health team's advice and make sure you're getting the proper treatment for your particular circumstances.

Making It Less Likely for Cancer to Return

Intermittent fasting has been shown to have a positive effect on whether or not cancer returns after it's treated. This is especially important because metastatic breast cancer, the most advanced type, typically shows up months or years after a woman has already been through treatment for an early cancer diagnosis. Only about 22 percent of women with metastatic breast cancer, also called stage IV breast cancer, live five years after diagnosis. The average life expectancy after diagnosis is three years.

Because there isn't a cure for metastatic breast cancer, preventing the cancer's recurrence becomes even more important. A 2016 study in *JAMA Oncology* looked at the effects of prolonged nightly fasting on breast cancer prognosis. The researchers found that women with early stage breast cancer who fasted for thirteen hours or more every night were 36 percent less likely to have cancer recurrence than women who fasted for less than thirteen hours nightly.

It All Comes Down to Autophagy

Your body is full of proteins and organelles that eventually become dysfunctional or die. This is a normal result of everyday living. But if these dead or damaged structures aren't cleared out from your body, they can lead to cell death, contribute to poor organ and tissue function, and even become cancerous.

This is where autophagy comes in. Autophagy, the major underlying mechanism behind the health benefits of intermittent fasting, means "self" (*auto*) "eating" (*phagy*). During autophagy, your body marks damaged cells, unused proteins, and other waste products in the body as junk. These damaged parts are then flagged and cleared out.

Autophagy also decreases chronic inflammation and supports natural immunity. Research shows that people with dysregulated autophagy are usually overweight, sleep more often, have higher cholesterol levels, and experience reduced brain function.

If autophagy is never stimulated to its full potential, dead and damaged cells and proteins can accumulate in your body and create all sorts of chronic health problems, such as Alzheimer's disease. Because they are never cleared from the body, dead proteins travel to the brain and get stuck there, contributing to the formation of the characteristic plaques associated with the disease. Abnormal autophagy has also been connected to obesity, diabetes, nutrient deficiencies, liver disease, atherosclerosis and heart disease, and cancer.

Fasting is one of the most effective ways to stimulate autophagy. You can also stimulate autophagy through a ketogenic diet and exercise, but these methods usually don't have as significant of an effect as intermittent fasting.

Why Women Are More Sensitive to Fasting

Now that you have a good grasp on the basics of intermittent fasting, the next step is understanding what makes women more sensitive to fasting than men. Like many issues related to female health, it really all comes down to hormones, which signal the molecules that regulate everything from your appetite to your sleeping habits to your sex drive. Your body has about fifty hormones, and keeping these delicate messengers in balance and harmony is critical to your well-being.

In this chapter, you'll learn what hormones are, what they do in your body, and how your stress levels can affect them. You'll also explore the different kinds of stress—good stress and bad stress—and why it's important to get your stress levels under control *before* you start intermittent fasting.

What Are Hormones?

To fully understand why women are more sensitive to fasting than men, you will need a little background on hormones and why they're important. Hormones are often called the body's chemical messengers. They're secreted into your blood, where they then travel to your organs and cells to perform their specific functions.

Hormones play roles in:

- Metabolic processes
- Reproduction and growth
- Sexual function
- Water and electrolyte balance
- Cognitive function and mood
- Hunger, thirst, and body temperature

There are around fifty hormones, and both women and men have them all, but what differs between the sexes are the hormone production sites, their concentration in the blood, and how they interact with different organs and systems. For example, both women and men have estrogen and testosterone, but as a general rule, women have more estrogen and men have more testosterone. This makes a huge difference in what goes on in the body and in how men and women respond to stressors and life experiences, like fasting.

Women's Reproductive Hormones

All hormones are important, but there are specific hormones in women that really steal the show, especially when discussing why women are more sensitive to fasting. Some of the hormones that play the biggest role in a woman's health—and whether or not you'll have positive results when fasting—are:

- **Estrogen:** One of a woman's two main sex hormones. It helps control your menstrual cycle, plays a vital role in reproduction, protects bone health, keeps cholesterol levels under control, and affects your heart, skin, and brain (including your mood).
- **Progesterone:** The other main sex hormone. It regulates your menstrual cycle, prepares your body for conception, and controls your sexual desire. Progesterone levels rise in the second half of your menstrual cycle.
- **Testosterone:** Testosterone is the main male sex hormone, but women have it too (in smaller amounts). In women, testosterone contributes to bone strength, maintains ovarian function, and plays a role in sexual health and desire. In order for your ovaries to work normally, you must have the proper balance of estrogen and testosterone.
- **Gonadotropin-releasing hormone (GnRH):** GnRH is classified as a releasing hormone. It acts on the pituitary gland, signaling it to make and release luteinizing hormone (LH) and follicle-stimulating hormone (FSH).
- **Luteinizing hormone (LH):** LH is released by the pituitary gland. It helps regulate your menstrual cycle and triggers ovulation, or the release of an egg from the ovary. LH levels are highest just before you ovulate.

- **Follicle-stimulating hormone (FSH):** FSH regulates your menstrual cycle and triggers the growth of eggs in your ovaries. FSH levels are highest right before ovulation.

When it comes to women, the major concern with intermittent fasting is that it can disrupt one or all of these crucial hormones, leading to infertility or trouble conceiving.

The Monthly Hormonal Cycle

During your reproductive years, your hormone levels rise and fall predictably throughout your monthly menstrual cycle (assuming your cycle is normal, of course). It works like this:

- **Day 1:** Low levels of estrogen and progesterone signal the pituitary gland to produce and release follicle-stimulating hormone (FSH). FSH starts the process of maturing a follicle, the sac in the ovary that contains the egg. During this process estrogen levels begin to rise. This is the first day of your period.
- **Days 2–11 (on average):** Estrogen levels start to rise as follicles (which contain eggs) develop on the ovaries. Around days 5–7, one follicle keeps growing, while the others stop. Estrogen levels continue to rise and, by day 8, period bleeding stops. Your uterine lining starts to build back up again.
- **Days 12–14 (on average):** Ovulation begins. The increased estrogen levels trigger the pituitary gland to release luteinizing hormone (LH). The release of LH causes the follicle to release an egg.
- **Days 15–22 (on average):** The follicle secretes estrogen and progesterone to prepare the body for pregnancy. Levels of estrogen and progesterone hormones rise, while levels of FSH and LH drop.
- **Days 23–28 (on average):** If the egg is not fertilized, levels of estrogen and progesterone begin to drop and continue dropping until the end of the menstrual cycle.

Every step of this cycle relies on the proper functioning of the step and hormone before it. If one of the hormones doesn't do its job correctly, then it can create a cascade, like a domino effect, that throws the entire cycle off.

The Effects of "Starving" on Reproductive Hormones

The reason some people think intermittent fasting is a bad idea for women is because of the potential for it to disrupt the complex workings of reproductive hormones. Women's bodies were physiologically designed to carry babies, and the process of developing a fetus is extremely calorie- and nutrient-demanding. That's why women are much more sensitive to potential starvation than men.

If your body senses impending starvation, or you're not getting enough calories or nutrients, it can respond by shutting down the reproductive system and doing whatever it can to prevent conception. That's because survival becomes the most important goal and reproduction falls way down the list of priorities. But how exactly does the body shut down reproduction? Through hormones. When a woman's body thinks there's a potential risk of starvation, it will respond by increasing the production of ghrelin and reducing the production of leptin, the two "hunger hormones" discussed in Chapter 1. The intent behind these hormonal changes is to make you feel hungry and force you to eat.

The decrease in leptin also causes the levels of another hormone called kisspeptin to go down. Kisspeptin, which is made in the hypothalamus of the brain, controls the entire cascade of reproductive hormones that leads to ovulation. A few studies show that women with less kisspeptin in their blood during early pregnancy may be at a higher risk of miscarriage or preeclampsia, a dangerous condition some women experience during pregnancy.

The Hypothalamic-Pituitary-Gonadal (HPG) Axis

To understand how impending starvation can translate to infertility, you need a little background on the hypothalamic-pituitary-gonadal (HPG) axis, which acts as the control board for reproduction. It's a four-step process:

1. Kisspeptin travels to the pituitary gland and triggers the release of gonadotropin-releasing hormone (GnRH).
2. The hypothalamus sends out GnRH.
3. GnRH signals the pituitary gland to release luteinizing hormone (LH) and follicle-stimulating hormone (FSH).
4. LH and FSH trigger the production of estrogen and progesterone and the release of an egg.

If kisspeptin levels are low, or kisspeptin isn't functioning correctly, it can halt this process, stopping a woman's menstrual cycle and causing infertility or making it difficult to conceive. And since intermittent fasting requires that you skip meals, some experts think that a woman's body will interpret it as impending starvation and shut off kisspeptin production.

But there's something important to note: This theory was developed after some small studies showed that fasting could negatively affect reproduction in female rats. There haven't been many human studies done to make any definitive statements about whether or not this happens in women. What's more, most of these studies used a form of intermittent fasting called alternate-day fasting where food and calories were completely restricted for a full twenty-four hours every other day. This fasting approach is way too intense for most women and not typically recommended, especially in the early stages of fasting.

There *have*, however, been studies on intermittent fasting and polycystic ovary syndrome (PCOS). Researchers from these studies have discovered that different types of fasting, including alternate-day fasting, twice-weekly fasting, and periodic fasting, can level out glucose and insulin and reduce excess testosterone in women. These hormonal changes actually have beneficial effects on ovary function and infertility in women with PCOS.

The Effect of Calorie Restriction

When it comes to concerns about hormonal imbalances and infertility, it's important to understand the difference between intermittent fasting and calorie restriction. As the name implies, calorie restriction forces you to reduce the overall amount of calories you're eating. You can eat at any time, but you can't go over a certain number of calories. *Intermittent fasting* is defined as "time-restricted feeding." There are no rules about how many calories you eat, just when you eat them. If you're following a well-balanced intermittent fasting schedule, there's a good chance you're not actually restricting the amount of calories you eat, just the period of time in which you eat them.

This is an important distinction because many people think that intermittent fasting is just a fancy or complicated way to restrict your overall calorie intake, but that's not the case. And thankfully so. Studies show that calorie restriction can actually lead to hormonal imbalances like decreased estrogen and thyroid hormones and problems with leptin. If this happens, it can cause related problems like:

- Weight gain/yo-yoing weight
- Intense hunger
- Loss of period and ovulation
- Infertility
- Weaker bones
- Mood changes and depression
- Constipation
- Difficulty sleeping and/or insomnia

In addition to hormonal imbalances and potential nutrient deficiencies, calorie restriction can:

- Make you really tired
- Reduce your metabolism (or your basal metabolic rate)
- Trigger the loss of lean muscle mass
- Negatively affect your immune system
- Increase stress and put you in a consistently bad mood
- Decrease concentration and negatively affect memory
- Trigger binge eating

The other problem is that when you're restricting calories, you increase your risk of developing nutrient deficiencies. The less food you eat, the fewer chances you have to get all of the vitamins and minerals you need. And if you're eating processed food and empty calories, the risk goes up even more.

On the other hand, a well-designed intermittent fasting plan has been shown to have a beneficial effect on hormonal imbalances and improve symptoms of various health conditions.

Hormonal Changes During Menopause

Menopause marks the end of your reproductive years, and there are actually three major stages to this transitional period: perimenopause, menopause, and postmenopause.

- *Perimenopause* can start ten years before menopause, but the average duration is three to four years. During perimenopause, you ovulate less so you experience fluctuating hormone levels and produce less progesterone. This change can lead to erratic or skipped periods.
- *Menopause* is the point when you no longer menstruate. You've officially reached menopause when you haven't had a monthly period for twelve consecutive months. During menopause, estrogen production in the ovaries almost completely stops. Because of this, you have lower levels of estrogen, as well as a lack of progesterone. The diminished hormone levels are the cause of the uncomfortable symptoms of menopause that many women experience.
- *Postmenopause* is the official name for the rest of your life after menopause. At this point, your ovaries no longer produce estrogen or progesterone. Any uncomfortable menopausal symptoms typically go away, but your risk of certain conditions, like osteoporosis, heart disease, and diabetes, rises. You may also notice changes in your skin tone and texture.

The concerns around intermittent fasting and hormone disruptions are generally geared toward premenopausal and perimenopausal women. Once you've reached the postmenopausal state, fasting's effects on estrogen are no longer a big concern. Actually, at this stage of life, fasting can become even more beneficial.

Estrogen helps your body properly utilize insulin. When you've reached menopause, and your ovaries no longer produce estrogen, you become less sensitive to its effects. As a result, your insulin levels can rise and your blood sugar levels can fluctuate, leading to weight gain, especially around your belly, and an increased risk of developing insulin resistance. But intermittent fasting can combat this, helping to control insulin and blood sugar and making it easier for you to manage your weight.

Signs of a Hormonal Imbalance

When hormones are in perfect balance, everything in your body is working as it should and you feel good. However, if hormones become unbalanced, it can lead to health problems and uncomfortable symptoms. Because hormones are involved in so many body processes, even a slight imbalance can have wide-ranging effects.

Some of the signs of a hormonal imbalance in women include:

- Bloating
- Irritability
- Heavy or irregular periods
- Vaginal dryness
- Inflammation in the vaginal walls
- Pain during sex
- Night sweats
- Thinning hair and/or hair loss
- Increased hair growth on the face
- Darkening of the skin
- Skin tags
- Weight gain and/or trouble losing weight
- Acne
- Blurred vision
- Increased sensitivity to cold and heat
- Dry skin
- Puffy face
- Bowel problems like constipation and/or diarrhea
- Changes in heart rate

- Sudden weight loss
- Frequent urination
- Muscle weakness
- Muscle aches and pains
- Pain, stiffness, and swelling in the joints
- Depression
- Anxiety
- Increased sweating
- Prominent stretch marks, usually purple or pink in color
- Increased hunger
- Fatty hump between the shoulders, sometimes called a buffalo hump

Things That Disrupt Hormones

Hormones are essential to good health and survival. The problem is, they can be really sensitive. If you're relying on sugar and caffeine for energy, stressing out all day, eating late at night, and going to bed after midnight—all things that can negatively affect your hormones—there's an excellent chance you have a hormonal imbalance.

Common diet and lifestyle habits that can disrupt a woman's hormones include:

- Eating late at night
- Eating a lot of sugar
- Too much stress
- Not getting enough sleep
- Drinking too much coffee
- Nutrient deficiencies
- An unhealthy diet
- Lack of regular exercise
- Using toxic beauty and cleaning products
- Using certain plastics

And if you're not careful about your approach, there's the potential that intermittent fasting can earn a spot on that list too. That's why you may have heard people say that women shouldn't do intermittent fasting. But that's not necessarily true. If you ease into it, listen to your body's signals, and do it right, intermittent fasting can actually be a great way to keep your hormones balanced. You just have to get your stress levels (and hormones) under control first.

What Is Stress?

Stress has been defined as "the nonspecific response of the body to any demand for change." The term, and definition, was coined in 1936 by Hans Selye, an endocrinologist, or hormone doctor, who was studying how certain factors, now called stressors, could affect human physiology.

At the time, most people believed that diseases were caused by bacteria, viruses, or other harmful pathogens. But Selye made a groundbreaking discovery when he found that exposing animals to different types of physical and emotional stimuli, like loud noises, bright lights, or unrelenting frustration, could actually change their physiology. When exposed to these stressors for an extended period of time, the animals started to experience physical changes, like enlarged adrenal glands and stomach ulcers, as well as chronic diseases, like heart attack, stroke, and even arthritis.

After more digging into stress over the years, researchers discovered that a lot of these health problems arise due to hormonal changes and resulting inflammation caused by stress. The stress response affects a number of hormones, including:

- Cortisol
- Catecholamines—epinephrine (adrenaline), norepinephrine (noradrenaline), and dopamine
- Vasopressin
- Gonadotropins—luteinizing hormone (LH) and follicle-stimulating hormone (FSH)
- Thyroid hormones
- Growth hormone
- Prolactin
- Insulin
- Estrogen and progesterone

The Type of Stress Matters

Stress is a broad term that can apply to a wide range of circumstances and stimuli. Sometimes the stress response can be lifesaving, while other times it can break down your body and make you more susceptible to sickness and disease. The main differentiator between which camp stress falls into depends on how long it lasts.

The two main types of stress are:

1. **Acute stress:** Acute stress is short-term stress that goes away as quickly as it comes. For example, when a car cuts you off and you slam on your brakes, the feeling that follows is acute stress. Once the stressor (the fear of a car accident) is gone and you calm down, the stress goes away and your hormones return to normal. But this kind of stress caused you to react in a certain way (slamming on your brakes) that could have saved your life, or at least protected you from injury.

2. **Chronic stress:** Chronic stress is stress that lasts for weeks, months, or even years. Chronic stress can have negative effects on your hormones that persist even after the stressor is removed. For example, if you finally leave a toxic romantic relationship after several years, it can take a few years for your hormones to normalize. If you don't get chronic stress under control, it can actually lead to health problems, like anxiety, depression, chronic headaches, weight gain, and digestive troubles.

As a whole, the word *stress* usually has negative connotations, but some types of stress are actually beneficial to your health.

Good versus Bad Stress

The goal isn't to get rid of all stress. Rather, the goal is to make sure your body interprets the stress in your life as good stress. But what's the difference? And why does it matter?

Stress is divided into two categories based on how it affects you physically, mentally, and physiologically. Good stress, technically referred to as eustress, is a mild to moderate level of stress that is ultimately beneficial. Eustress motivates you to pursue a goal, overcome a hurdle, and/or reach a desired outcome. When you reach that goal, the stress goes away and you usually experience happiness, contentment, excitement, and inspiration. Eustress can increase resilience and improve physical strength. Examples of eustress include:

- Working toward a deadline
- Practicing for an upcoming performance
- Training for an athletic game or event

On the other hand, bad stress, also called distress, is chronic, unrelenting stress that never seems to go away. Instead of motivating you to work toward your goals, distress leads to overwhelming feelings and makes it harder to achieve what you set out to do. Distress can hinder productivity, interfere with daily life, and cause health problems, like weight gain, depression, and increased susceptibility to colds and the flu. Examples of distress include:

- Constant work deadlines
- Toxic romantic relationships or friendships
- Trauma or death in the family

Fasting Is a Form of Stress

One of the best examples of good stress is exercise. Exercise is technically classified as a stressor to your muscles and cardiovascular system, but ultimately, this type of stress makes both of these systems stronger (as long as you don't overdo it and you give yourself enough time to recover after particularly intense sessions).

Dr. Mark Mattson of Johns Hopkins University explains that intermittent fasting puts stress on your body in the same way that exercise does. When you abstain from food for a certain period of time, it puts your body's cells under mild stress. Over time, your cells learn to cope with this stress and respond to it in a better way. And when your body is better at dealing with stress, it has an increased ability to resist illness and disease. But there's a caveat.

Whether or not fasting works as a good stressor or a bad stressor depends on your overall stress load—or how many total stressors you have in your life. And here's where it gets trickier: The American Institute of Stress points out that it's really hard to define stress and make clear distinctions between what classifies as eustress or distress because stress is extremely subjective.

Because everyone reacts differently to certain things and has different perspectives and mindsets, the line between good stress and bad stress can become blurred. Some women interpret a difficult task as a welcome challenge, while other women presented with the same task get immediately overwhelmed. In other words, what's good stress to one woman may be bad stress to another woman. And typically, your interpretation of stress, and your body's physiological response to it, all comes down to your overall stress load.

Stress Overload

Your overall stress load is the total amount of stressors you're currently dealing with. Someone with one or two life stressors has a low stress load, while someone who seems to be dodging stressful event after stressful event is either under, or on their way to, stress overload.

Simply put, stress overload means you're dealing with too much stress. At this point, it doesn't matter whether an individual stressor would be classified as good stress or bad stress. When you have too many stressors in your life—or you have poor stress management skills—your body physiologically interprets every form of stress as bad stress.

A study published in the *International Journal of Stress Management* divided the symptoms of poor stress management into six major clusters. Here are some signs you're dealing with too much stress:

- **Body complaints:** body aches, itchiness, fatigue, body weakness, reduced libido, teeth grinding and/or clenching.
- **Gastrointestinal disturbances:** stomach pains, nausea, skin rashes, acne, vomiting, and diarrhea.
- **Respiratory problems:** stuffy or runny nose, sore throat, frequent sneezing, and earaches.
- **Moodiness:** waking up feeling unrested, increased irritability, emotional outbursts, impatience, muscle tics or twitches, increased anger, anxiety, depression, and abuse of alcohol or drugs to cope.
- **Nervous habits:** increased nervousness, compulsiveness, pacing, making frequent mistakes, nail-biting, and trembling.
- **Cognitive disruption:** difficulty focusing, indecisiveness, and forgetfulness.

A good way to figure out whether you have too much stress is to ask yourself some basic questions. Do you feel challenged but motivated? Do you feel productive and accomplished when you hit your goals? If so, you probably have normal levels of stress. Do you feel overwhelmed, withdrawn, and tired? Are you irritable, moody, and having trouble being productive? If so, you could be dealing with stress overload.

Before starting with intermittent fasting, it's important to evaluate how well you are managing the stress in your life. If you've determined that you are in a state of stress overload, your number one goal should be to manage that stress and get yourself back to a normal physiological state. Then you will be ready to begin intermittent fasting.

The Effects of Fasting Stress on Women

If you don't bring your overall stress load down before you try to throw intermittent fasting into the mix, there's a much higher chance that you'll run into problems. Instead of providing the myriad of health benefits that it's known for and increasing your resilience, fasting could become the metaphorical straw that broke the camel's back, creating a negative energy balance that can affect all of your interconnected hormones.

It's not the fasting itself that's a problem. It's the combination of too many stressors with the addition of another stressor: fasting. On its own, fasting is a good stressor that helps your body adapt and improve physically and mentally. But when combined with a bunch of other things that you're either physically or psychologically interpreting as bad stress, it could send your cortisol response through the roof.

As a result, your body's production of gonadotropin-releasing hormone goes down and your ovaries stop producing the right amounts of estrogen and progesterone. At the same time, your body is using progesterone to keep up with your cortisol demand, which further unbalances your estrogen levels. If this goes on too long, your fertility can be affected.

How the Stress Response Works

To grasp the connection between stress and reproduction, you need to understand how the stress response works. At its core is the hypothalamic-pituitary-adrenal (HPA) axis. The HPA axis is the connection between your hypothalamus (H), pituitary glands (P), and adrenal glands (A). Its job is to handle your body's reaction to stress.

When something stressful happens, the sympathetic nervous system releases two neurotransmitters and hormones: epinephrine (adrenaline) and norepinephrine (noradrenaline). Aside from constricting your blood vessels and increasing your heart rate, these hormones kick your HPA axis into gear. In response to epinephrine and norepinephrine:

- The hypothalamus sends out corticotropin-releasing hormone (CRH).
- CRH travels to the pituitary gland, where it triggers the release of adrenocorticotropic hormone (ACTH).
- ACTH moves to the adrenal cortex, where it tells the adrenal glands to release cortisol, the main stress hormone.

The point of all of this is to get your body ready to either fight the stressor or run from it. It's the foundation of fight-or-flight mode. When your stress levels are high, you are in prime shape to fight off an attack or flee from one. Blood is pumping to your legs, your eyesight improves, and you become extra vigilant—all thanks to hormones.

If the stressor goes away, these hormones will remain elevated for a few hours, but then they'll eventually return to normal and you'll go back into parasympathetic mode—the physiological state where your nervous system is relaxed and you feel calm.

That all sounds great and helpful, but for many women, unmanaged stress interrupts that cycle. Because the stressors never actually go away, stress levels remain elevated, which means the hormones remain elevated, and your body has to compensate to find a way to maintain the abnormally high hormone levels for days, weeks, or even years.

The Problems with Cortisol

Although there are several hormones involved in the stress response, cortisol is nicknamed "the stress hormone" because it plays a primary role in activating your fight-or-flight response. Once cortisol is released into your bloodstream, it triggers a large surge in glucose that supplies fast-acting and immediate energy to your large muscles, like your legs. This puts you in a position where you can run really fast if you choose the flight option of the stress response.

Cortisol also lowers the production and release of insulin so that glucose remains available for use instead of getting stored, and it narrows your blood vessels and arteries so that your blood pumps harder, supplying the oxygen and nutrients you might need to respond to a potential threat.

In addition to making your body the perfect machine for handling an immediate threat, normal levels of cortisol:

- Help control blood sugar levels
- Reduce inflammation
- Regulate metabolism
- Help with memory
- Support healthy pregnancies

During times of stress, blood levels of cortisol and other hormones involved in the stress response can increase by as much as two to five times. While this is okay in the short term, if the stress never goes away and the levels stay elevated for too long, it can cause a bunch of health problems, such as:

- Changes in your menstrual cycle
- Reduced libido
- Weight gain and obesity
- Suppression of the immune system
- Chronic inflammation
- Heart disease
- Thyroid disease
- Chronic fatigue syndrome
- Blood sugar imbalances and increased risk of diabetes

If you throw intermittent fasting into an already stressful lifestyle, the chances of it negatively affecting cortisol levels increase.

Stress, Progesterone, and Estrogen

As we have seen, chronic stress can cause multiple health problems; it can also wreak havoc on your reproductive hormones. But before jumping into this, you need a little background on the relationship between progesterone and estrogen.

Progesterone and estrogen are complementary hormones; they perform opposite functions. For example:

- Estrogen increases body fat, while progesterone helps you use fat for energy.
- Estrogen makes you retain salt and fluid, while progesterone is a natural diuretic.
- Estrogen increases your sex drive, while progesterone decreases it.
- Estrogen impairs blood glucose, while progesterone helps normalize it.

The point is that each hormone has an opposite, but equal, reaction, so when they are in balance, you remain in balance. But when you're stressed, that balance gets thrown off significantly.

Progesterone is the precursor to cortisol. In other words, your body uses progesterone to make cortisol. If you're constantly stressed, your body needs to find ways to make cortisol to keep up with the demand, so it uses the progesterone in your blood. This lowers levels of progesterone and can lead to a progesterone deficiency that, in turn, leads to a hormonal imbalance called estrogen dominance.

What Is Estrogen Dominance?

Estrogen dominance is a fancy way of saying that your progesterone levels are low and your estrogen levels are high. When you're estrogen dominant, estrogen is basically running a show that's supposed to be an equally balanced duet between progesterone and estrogen. It's like progesterone has left the building and estrogen is now forced to do a job it doesn't know how to do on its own. And when that happens, things can get messed up pretty quickly.

Some signs of estrogen dominance are:

- Mood swings and irritability
- Worsening PMS symptoms, like tender breasts, headaches, acne, and mood swings
- Irregular or heavy menstrual periods
- Decreased libido
- Bloating
- Weight gain
- Hair loss
- Difficulty sleeping
- Anxiety and/or panic attacks
- Brain fog and memory problems
- Hot flashes and/or night sweats
- Low energy and fatigue
- Fertility issues

Excess estrogen also makes your brain more sensitive to ghrelin (the hormone that tells you you're hungry) and less sensitive to leptin (the hormone that tells you you're full). So if your levels of estrogen are high all the time, there's a good chance you always feel hungry. And that's a situation that can make intermittent fasting extremely difficult.

The good news is that once your estrogen levels are balanced, these symptoms will likely go away and you might be surprised to find that you feel satisfied even during your fasting times.

Stress and Insulin

During times of stress, one of your body's priorities is to make sure that you have enough energy to handle whatever's about to come your way. And to your body, sugar (glucose) equals energy.

To ensure that you have adequate glucose levels to handle the stress response, insulin levels drop and epinephrine and glucagon rise to facilitate release of glucose from the liver. While this is happening, cortisol and growth hormone levels also increase, making your muscle and fat tissues less sensitive to insulin. The goal of this process is to make more glucose available in your bloodstream so you can fight or run.

But if you're feeling stressed when you're sitting at your computer or on the couch watching *Netflix*, and not using up that glucose (by running away from your threat), this cascade of events can lead to stress-induced hyperglycemia (high blood sugar) and even the development of insulin resistance, in both the short and long term.

While many people are aware of the detrimental effects that chronic stress can have on the body, what's less well known and perhaps more interesting is that these effects can be seen with acute stress too. In one animal study published in the *Journal of Endocrinology* in 2013, researchers found that even short-term stress can diminish the liver's response to insulin and negatively affect how the body metabolizes glucose—the hallmark characteristics of insulin resistance.

This finding shines the spotlight of the importance for women to not only find ways to manage chronic stress, but to figure out how to react more positively to acute stressors as well.

Other Hormones Affected by Stress

Cortisol, estrogen, progesterone, and insulin are important hormones involved in the stress response, but they're not the only ones. Stress also affects:

- **Thyroid hormones (T3, T4, TSH, and calcitonin):** Your thyroid and reproductive hormones are intricately connected. And just like stress can interfere with your reproductive hormones directly, it can also interfere indirectly by negatively affecting your thyroid hormones. When you're stressed, your thyroid function gets downregulated. In other words, the thyroid lowers its production of TSH (thyroid-stimulating hormone), T3, and T4. This is actually a by-product of the effect of cortisol on your nervous system.
- **Ghrelin and leptin:** Stress can increase ghrelin and decrease leptin, making you feel hungry all the time. Of course, when this happens you tend to crave carb- or sugar-rich foods that aren't the best options. In a study that looked at stress's effect on appetite, researchers found that approximately 78 percent of stressed women craved sweets. As a result, these stressed women also tended to have larger bellies.
- **Growth hormone:** Growth hormone (GH) enhances your metabolism, contributes to the development of lean muscle mass, and helps you maintain a healthy body weight. During times of acute physical stress, levels of GH in your body increase. But when you're chronically emotionally or psychologically stressed, GH can actually decrease.
- **Vasopressin:** Vasopressin is a pituitary hormone that's involved in water retention and blood pressure control. Stress can cause a rapid

release of vasopressin that leads to high blood pressure and water weight gain.

- **Prolactin:** Prolactin is the main pituitary hormone involved in breast milk production, but it also has three hundred other functions in your body. When you're stressed, prolactin levels increase. While this could be a good thing if you're nursing, if you're not, it can lead to menstrual disturbances, unwanted milk production, and low estrogen.

Unmanaged stress can have implications for every system in your body. That's why it's vitally important to get your stress levels under control before you attempt to throw another stressor, even if it's a potentially good stressor like intermittent fasting, into the mix.

Fasting and the Nervous System

Some studies have shown that fasting may affect the nervous systems of men and women differently. In a 2016 study done with men, fasting increased parasympathetic activity of the nervous system. In other words, fasting settled the nervous system and stress response down, making the men feel calmer. In a 2017 study done with women, fasting kicked the sympathetic nervous system into higher gear. In other words, women became more stressed and entered into a fight-or-flight state.

These studies have prompted the argument that fasting is bad for women and can increase stress and anxiety. However, it's extremely important to note that both of these studies used a forty-eight-hour water-only fast. That means that the participants ate nothing for two whole days. It's also important to note that the men in the first study were amateur weight lifters in decent physical shape while the women in the second study were overweight and had elevated levels of perceived stress.

The proper conclusion here would be that water-only fasting isn't a good idea for stressed-out overweight women. Intermittent fasting after getting your stress levels under control is a totally different ball game.

Women Are More Stressed Than Men

In addition to the unique way that a woman's body responds to stress, when it comes to overall life experience, women are generally more negatively affected by stress than men. According to the American Psychological Association:

- Women are more likely than men to report feeling a lot of stress.
- Almost 50 percent of women say their stress has increased over the past five years, compared to 39 percent of men.
- Women are more likely to experience physical and emotional symptoms of stress, like headache, stomachache, and/or sadness.
- Married women report feeling more stressed than single women.

Why the stress discrepancy between men and women? One of the biggest reasons is that, in general, women tend to do more domestic (unpaid) labor—about 37 percent more—than men. In addition to possibly working outside of the home, women often shoulder a larger portion of responsibilities for cooking, cleaning, childcare, and making sure the home life is running smoothly.

Another reason for gender differences in stress levels is that women are often more likely than men to try to force emotions that aren't necessarily in line with what they're feeling—a characteristic that's been deemed "emotional labor." For example, research shows that when a woman is in a leadership role at work, she will feign optimism, calmness, and empathy, even if she is truly feeling overwhelmed and frazzled. Hiding your true emotions can be not only stressful but also downright exhausting.

Women also have been traditionally more likely to put pressure on themselves to be well liked or to live up to a certain ideal, whereas men are generally less concerned with being nice or liked by everyone around them. On the flip side, men are more likely to engage in activities that help them manage their stress, like playing sports or listening to music.

Of course, these are generalities, and gender norms evolve as the world changes: Many men are doing more work around the house, for example. Nonetheless, statistics and research into male and female behavior patterns do support the fact that women tend to be more significantly affected by stress.

Women Have Higher Nutrient Needs

Some concern around intermittent fasting comes from the fact that women have higher needs for certain nutrients, like iron, folate, and calcium, than men. Some people worry that if you're not eating as often, you'll be putting yourself at risk of developing nutrient deficiencies, but that's why it's important to emphasize that fasting doesn't necessarily mean you're eating less food. It only means you're eating within a shorter window of time.

You can still eat the same volume of food and the same number of calories. That choice is yours. And as long as you're focusing on optimizing your nutrient intake by eating a variety of fresh, whole foods at every meal, you have nothing to worry about in that area. In fact, some women who eat all day and into the night can actually have a higher risk of developing nutrient deficiencies if they're eating highly processed foods that are full of carbs, sugar, and artificial ingredients but empty of any real nutrients.

What you don't want to do, however, is combine fasting with a standard American diet that's full of processed foods and carbohydrates. While there aren't any specific "food rules" or prohibitions connected to intermittent fasting, it is beneficial to change your diet to some degree. You don't have to count calories, but if you're trying to reach some pretty lofty health goals, you'll have to put in the extra work. Intermittent fasting is an excellent tool for improving your health, but it's not a miracle solution.

Stress Relief First, Intermittent Fasting Second

When you picked up this book, you may not have expected such an in-depth lesson on stress and hormones. But knowing how everything works is critical to understanding why women can be more sensitive to fasting than men, and why some people are under the false impression that absolutely no woman should fast, no matter what.

The key to making intermittent fasting a positive experience for you is to make stress relief and hormonal balance your first priority. If you're under chronic distress, you need to get that under control before you incorporate intermittent fasting into your routine. Because intermittent fasting is an additional stressor, it can contribute to chronic stress and the excessive production and release of cortisol. Normalizing your cortisol levels and ensuring that your adrenal glands are working properly should be your main focus before you add fasting to the mix.

Once your stress levels are under control and your hormones are back in balance, intermittent fasting then becomes a form of eustress (positive, beneficial stress) that can push you toward achieving your health goals.

Even though you may be eager to jump into intermittent fasting right away, especially after learning about all of the benefits, doing so can do more harm than good if you're too stressed to begin with. Luckily, there are many changes you can make—many of which are quite simple—to get your stress and hormones under control so that you can start fasting as soon as your body is ready.

Getting a Handle on Stress and Hormones

If you're considering intermittent fasting, your first priority should be getting your stress levels under control and balancing your hormones. You may be eager to start an intermittent fasting schedule right away, but putting your initial effort and focus into stress management greatly reduces the risk that you'll experience any negative effects from fasting. This chapter covers all of the different things you can do to get your stress levels and hormones under control before you begin intermittent fasting.

If you have a pretty good handle on your stress levels and don't have any signs of a hormonal imbalance, you can start slowly with intermittent fasting and see how it goes. If you notice negative changes instead of positive ones, you always have the option to scale back or try a different form of intermittent fasting until you find the schedule that works best for you. But even if you feel like your stress levels are under control right now, these stress management and hormone-balancing techniques are a great way to ensure they stay that way.

Signs You Need to Start with Hormone Balancing

Stress is a normal part of life. There's no way to *completely* get rid of it, so having stressors in your life doesn't automatically make you a bad candidate for intermittent fasting. That being said, there's a thin line between stress and burnout.

If you have too much stress or you're constantly overworked, there's a good chance that your hormones are suffering, and if that's the case, you need to alleviate your burnout and get your hormones in order before you do anything else. So, how do you know where you stand? You listen to your body.

Regular stress can help motivate you to get up and get things done, but too much stress can lead to burnout. If you experience a handful of the following symptoms regularly, you need to put intermittent fasting on the back burner for now. Instead, your first priority needs to be stress management.

- Chronic fatigue
- Feeling emotionally drained
- Trouble sleeping/insomnia
- Forgetfulness
- Inability to concentrate
- Having a hard time completing tasks
- Short attention span
- Frequent illness or infections
- Loss of appetite
- Tension, worry, and/or anxiety

- Depression
- Irritability and/or lack of patience
- Anger and/or angry outbursts
- Loss of enjoyment
- Negative self-talk
- Pessimism
- Isolation
- Feelings of disconnectedness
- Feelings of apathy
- Physical symptoms, like shortness of breath, dizziness, chest pain, and frequent headaches

Make sure you get any physical symptoms checked out by a doctor.

Prioritizing Stress Management

One of the problems with burnout is that you feel like you don't have enough time to do *anything*. So when it comes to self-care, you can forget about it. But here's something that you need to understand: Stress management and self-care are not luxuries; they're necessities. If you're not taking the time to do things that help reduce your stress levels, you're going to burn out.

If you're already burned out, things will just get worse until you get in the driver's seat and take control of your stress, rather than continuing to let it control you. Just like you would schedule important work deadlines or sports games or playdates for your kids, you need to schedule and prioritize stress management for you.

Block off certain times in your calendar every day for stress management and self-care. Keep in mind that this doesn't mean that you have to take a two-hour bubble bath with flickering candles every night (although that would be nice). You just need some time each day to decompress and calm your nervous system. This could be a ten-minute meditation session in the morning before the kids wake up or thirty minutes of yoga during your lunch break.

Although there are proven ways to reduce your stress levels and balance your hormones, there's no one-size-fits-all answer to what stress management looks like for everyone. You have to learn the available techniques and experiment with different combinations of them to see what works best for you.

Do Yoga

You might hear the phrase "do yoga" and think of lithe bodies contorted into positions that look pretty stressful, but there's a lot of research that backs up yoga's beneficial effects on your stress levels and hormones.

In one study conducted by the Yoga Research Society and the Sidney Kimmel Medical College at Thomas Jefferson University, researchers found that after a fifty-minute yoga session, cortisol levels dropped significantly. Another study published in the *International Journal of Psychosomatics* looked at the effects of Hatha yoga on healthy women and found that this type of yoga could lower cortisol and prolactin, which can cause problems with estrogen and progesterone if levels get too high.

In addition to the physical effects, the women who were doing yoga regularly also had more life satisfaction and improved mood, while reporting fewer feelings of anger, excitability, and physical complaints, like aches and pains. They also became more extroverted and experienced improvements in learning how to cope with stress.

A main focus of many types of yoga is to slow down and focus on your breathing, which certainly helps with stress management. Some yoga poses that are particularly good for balancing hormones are:

- Rabbit Pose (*Sasangasana*)
- Cobra Pose (*Bhujangasana*)
- Camel Pose (*Ustrasana*)
- Fish Pose (*Matsyasana*)
- Garland Pose (*Malasana*)

Breath work, or pranayama, also helps to calm your mind and body.

Practice Meditation

Meditation helps reduce cortisol and increase DHEA, a hormone that can help improve the function of your adrenal glands. DHEA has also been connected to weight loss and better mood. Meditation physically changes the nerve pathways in your brain, making you more resilient to stress and helping to lower anxiety. In other words, meditation might not make the stress in your life go away, but it can help you deal with it in a more positive way. Meditation has also been shown to increase melatonin levels, so doing a quick meditation right before bed can help promote restful sleep, another thing that can help balance your hormones.

The good news is that there's no right or wrong way to meditate. So if your first thought when you hear the word *meditate* is "I can't," rest assured, you can. The point of meditation isn't to clear your mind of any and all thoughts; rather, you want to acknowledge your thoughts and feelings without judging them or labeling them as good or bad.

The even better news is that it doesn't require a huge time commitment. You can see significant benefits by meditating for just ten minutes a day. Consistency—meaning practicing every day—seems to be more important than duration—or the amount of time that you actually sit and meditate in one session.

If you're new to meditating, you can start by following along with a guided meditation. There are thousands available online (try *YouTube*) to help get you started.

Learn How to Breathe

Before you raise your eyebrow at the idea of learning how to breathe, consider this: Even though it's an involuntary action, most people don't breathe correctly. Humans are supposed to be belly breathers—meaning you take air in, expand your belly, and let air out. However, because of chronic stress and never being taught how to breathe properly, many people have turned into chest breathers—taking air into the chest in a short, shallow breath and then exhaling through the mouth.

This shallow breathing limits the range of motion of the diaphragm. As a result, the lower part of your lungs don't get enough oxygenated air, leaving you feeling short of breath and anxious. On the other hand, proper breathing techniques ensure that you have a full oxygen exchange—oxygen comes in and carbon dioxide goes out. This regulates your heart rate, reduces anxiety, stabilizes blood pressure, and lowers your cortisol levels. In fact, breathing is so important that there are several institutes and learning centers dedicated solely to teaching people how to breathe correctly.

If you're feeling wound up all the time, check in with your breathing and see if you're doing it right. Here's how to breathe properly:

1. Breathe in through your nose.
2. Fill your belly with air.
3. Breathe out through your nose.

On average, you take about 22,000 breaths each day. That's 22,000 opportunities to easily reduce stress and calm your nervous system.

Breathe Deeply

Practicing deep breathing is a powerful stress management tool. When you're stressed or anxious, your breathing becomes shallow and you may even hold your breath. If you're stressed all the time, this means that you're probably not getting the right amount of oxygen and your breathing is never properly telling your nervous system to relax.

Carve out some time to practice deep breathing for a few minutes each day. Deep breathing is especially helpful if you do it in the morning before you start your day and then again before falling asleep. You don't even have to get out of bed to do it!

Here's how to practice deep breathing:

1. Sit up straight or lie on your back in a comfortable spot. Put one hand on your chest and the other on your stomach.
2. Take a deep breath in through your nose, keeping your mouth closed. Let your belly fully expand with air and hold for a few seconds. The hand that's on your stomach should rise, but the hand that's on your chest shouldn't move very much.
3. Purse your lips as if you're about to whistle and exhale fully through your mouth, pushing out as much air as you can. The hand on your belly should come down until all of the air is gone.
4. Repeat steps 2 and 3 five to ten times or until you feel your body start to relax.

It's normal to feel a little dizzy as your body gets used to deep breathing, so don't be alarmed if this happens. That's why it's a good idea to be sitting or lying down when you do it. And make sure to take your time getting back into an upright position when you're done.

Keep a Journal

According to a study done by Harvard University in 2016, women are more likely to hold things in—and hold longer grudges—than men. You may think that keeping your feelings inside is a way to keep the peace, but while not speaking your mind may help you avoid external conflict, it creates a lot of internal conflict. If you aren't good at saying how you feel out loud, use a journal to get your thoughts and frustrations out. Research shows that doing this can reduce cortisol levels, simultaneously reducing stress and anxiety.

Once per day, sit down and make a list of everything that's stressing you out or worrying you. This can provide instant relief, like a weight has been lifted from your shoulders, and long-term relief, as hormone levels balance out. It's especially helpful if you're someone who lies awake all night worrying about your to-do list. Journaling helps get the thoughts out of your head and onto the paper, so you don't feel like you have to keep track of everything in your head.

If you're worried that someone will read thoughts or feelings that you don't want anyone to see, you can write them down in a computer document and then delete them or write them on a piece of paper and then tear it up or burn it. As long as you get the emotions out of your head and your body and onto paper, it can have positive effects on your stress and hormones.

In addition to writing down your worries, you should also make it a habit to write daily gratitude lists. Writing down three small (or big) things you're grateful for every day can help reduce stress levels and serve as a reminder of the positive things in your life.

Listen to Uplifting Music

You know that feeling you get when your favorite song comes on the radio? Turns out there's actual science behind how that works. Research shows that no matter what kind of mood you're in, listening to music that you enjoy can lower cortisol levels and help reduce stress. Music can also increase oxytocin, often called the love hormone, and decrease vasopressin, a hormone that can increase blood pressure.

In addition to the actual physical effects it has on your hormone levels, music also helps divert your attention away from ruminating on stress and incessant mind chatter, especially if you sing along.

While any music is beneficial, classical music seems to have the greatest effect. Studies show that classical music can help lower stress hormones and decrease your blood pressure, heart rate, and pulse.

Play some music when you're getting ready for work in the morning or turn on Spotify as you prepare and cook dinner. Dance and sing along and really try to get into it. Even if it's not your favorite music genre, it's a good idea to turn on a little classical music as you wind down before bed.

Call Out Your Negative Voice

Your brain has a propensity toward negativity—not necessarily because it wants to be a Debbie Downer, but it actually thinks that being negative is a way to protect you from possible threats. Your brain thinks that if you're always on alert and anticipating that something bad will happen, then you will be ready to fight and less likely to be caught off guard. This phenomenon—called the negativity bias—was extremely useful back when early humans needed it to survive in the wild. But nowadays, it's an unnecessary contributor to stress and anxiety.

That's where positive thinking and affirmations come in. These are powerful stress-reduction tools that can rewire the neurons in your brain and make it easier for you to think positively—a concept known as neuroplasticity. Positive affirmations also help balance your stress hormones.

And the more you engage in positive thinking and positive affirmations, the easier it becomes for you to naturally think positively. Every time you catch yourself thinking negative thoughts like "I'll never get all of this work done" or "I have no time to relax," try to replace those thoughts with positive ones like "I will finish everything I need to, one thing at a time" and "I will make time to relax, even just for ten minutes."

Training your brain in this way will be really helpful down the line when you're ready to start intermittent fasting. When you first begin intermittent fasting, you'll notice your brain naturally wants to go to negative thoughts like "This is too hard" or "I'm starving. I'll never make it through my fasting window." Pay attention when thoughts like these come up and counteract them by saying things like "My thoughts don't define me. I can and will succeed."

Prioritize Tasks and Avoid Procrastination

Procrastination may seem like a good idea in the moment, but really, you're just delaying the inevitable. Besides, it doesn't actually feel good. You may be sitting there outwardly looking like you're calmly scrolling through *Instagram*, but inside you're freaking out—or your hormones are at least—because you have a lot to do and you're not doing it.

When you procrastinate, it increases your cortisol levels and puts your amygdala (the part of your brain that's responsible for anxiety) on high alert. When your amygdala is constantly activated, you can't ever relax.

The catch-22 is that the more stressed you are, the more likely you are to procrastinate and put off tasks, even simple ones like dropping something off at the post office or responding to an email. So, while the advice to "just do it" comes from a good place, it's not always that simple for someone dealing with burnout.

When you have a lot on your plate, it's helpful to write out a manageable to-do list and focus only on that list for the day. Don't think about everything you have to get done this week or this month—just put your attention on that one day and try to stay focused enough to get through it. Starting with the more difficult tasks and then moving on to simpler tasks can be helpful too, since your brain is usually sharper in the morning, especially when you're dealing with chronic stress.

If you prioritize your tasks and focus on getting through your daily to-do lists as efficiently as possible, you'll start to notice that it feels like a weight is being lifted off your shoulders. When this happens, it gets easier to avoid procrastination.

Get Enough Sleep

Skimping on sleep is one of the worst things you can do for your health and your hormones. When you're sleep deprived, your body increases its production of ghrelin, the hormone that tells you you're hungry and it's time to get some food, and decreases its production of leptin, the hormone that tells your brain you're full. When ghrelin levels are high and leptin levels are low, you're pretty much hungry all the time.

Even if you're doing everything else right, a lack of sleep negatively affects your hormones, so it's really important to try to find a way to get enough sleep every night. Ideally, you should aim for eight hours of quality sleep each night. In addition to focusing on the amount of sleep you're getting, a regular sleep schedule—meaning you go to bed at the same time every night and wake up at the same time every morning—can help regulate your hormones.

It's also beneficial to be in bed, sleeping, by 10 p.m. This helps keep your circadian rhythm functioning normally, but also makes it easier to stick to your fasting schedule (when the time comes) because you'll be sleeping instead of watching TV on the couch, trying to talk yourself out of that bag of chips.

Create an Ideal Sleep Environment

If you're having trouble sleeping, changing up your sleep environment can do wonders. If there's light from an alarm clock or a full moon streaming through the window, loud noises, or constant interruption from pets trying to wake you up for their next meal, there's a slim chance you're going to sleep well through the night and wake up feeling great.

There are many things you can do to improve your sleep environment and most of them are small, easy changes. You can:

- Make sure the room is completely dark. Unplug electronics and get blackout curtains or wear a sleep mask to bed.
- Adjust the thermostat in your room to between 60°F and 67°F. The National Sleep Foundation says this is the best temperature for getting a good night's sleep.
- Get breathable cotton sheets so you don't wake up sweating.
- Lock your pets out of your bedroom until morning (this can be a tough one!).
- Wear socks to bed. Studies show that people who wear socks to bed fall asleep faster and stay sleeping longer than people who don't.
- If there are outside noises that you can't control, wear ear plugs or use a white noise machine or app.
- Invest in a comfortable, supportive mattress.
- Make sure your pillows are comfortable.

In addition to changing your sleep environment, you can also make some changes to your routine and how you approach bedtime:

- Avoid eating spicy foods with dinner.

- Turn off your phone and all electronics at least an hour before bedtime.
- Take a hot shower before bed.
- Listen to soft, relaxing music.
- Diffuse lavender or other relaxing essential oils, like valerian, cedarwood, or Roman chamomile.
- Spray lavender oil on your pillow or rub a little on your neck and behind your ears.
- Focus on your breathing and relaxing all of your muscles.

Reduce Your Caffeine Intake

Caffeine is a weird thing. On one hand, it can help stimulate autophagy, the foundation of most of the health benefits of intermittent fasting (see Chapter 1). On the other hand, it can spike your cortisol levels and contribute to adrenal gland dysfunction, especially if you're drinking too much caffeine.

Coffee, especially, can be a double-edged sword because it's one of the most pesticide-treated crops out there. If you're not drinking organic coffee, you could be exposing yourself to hormone-disrupting chemicals with every cup. And when you're working really hard to get your hormones under control so you can start fasting, that's the last thing you want to do.

If you're really stressed, it's best to avoid coffee and all other caffeine completely until your adrenal glands recover. Once you're feeling like yourself again, you can add some caffeine back in, but go slowly.

Most people do okay with 400 milligrams of caffeine per day, which is roughly the amount in 4 cups. Keep in mind, though, that a "cup" of coffee is really only 5–6 ounces, not 8—and definitely not 20, which is what you get when you order the largest size at many chain coffee shops.

If you're looking for a pick-me-up without the potential negative effects, get your caffeine from matcha green tea instead of coffee. Matcha is rich in L-theanine, an amino acid that helps your body process caffeine differently. As a result, you experience a calm alertness coupled with a sustained energy boost, instead of a jittery energy followed by a major crash.

Consider Stress-Supporting Supplements

Stress is so common that there are supplements designed specifically to help your body physically cope with it. As stress management concerns have become more mainstream, these supplements, often called adaptogens, have become increasingly popular.

Adding some of these adaptogens to your routine can help your body deal with stress and reduce the negative effects that stress overload and high cortisol levels can have on your health. They also have a physically calming effect. They're not like sedatives that can make you feel groggy; they provide just enough stress relief to take the edge off.

Here are some of the most common adaptogens:

- Ashwagandha
- Asian ginseng
- Holy basil (tulsi)
- Siberian ginseng
- Rhodiola
- Reishi mushroom
- Maca
- Milk thistle
- Astragalus

These adaptogens are available as teas, in powders that you can mix into smoothies, and as capsules. Some of the supplements contain a blend of different adaptogens that support your system in different but complementary ways.

If you do decide to start taking stress-supporting supplements, make sure you have a discussion with your doctor or a qualified nutritionist who can guide you down the right path and help you choose the best one(s) for you.

Support Your Digestive Health

Digestive ailments like constipation and diarrhea are really uncomfortable. Just fixing these problems is a great way to reduce your stress and make you feel lighter overall. But digestive health includes more than reducing symptoms. The bacteria that live in your gut actually play a huge role in hormone balance.

There's a collection of bacteria in your gut that's called the estrobolome. This collection of bacteria has a powerful effect on the amount of circulating estrogen in your blood. When the estrobolome is healthy and functioning properly, your estrogen levels are normal. But when your gut environment is unhealthy, it can lead to either too much or too little estrogen. This can cause problems with weight, mood, and libido.

Gut bacteria also regulate melatonin (which is connected to sleep), thyroid hormones, and norepinephrine and epinephrine, two hormones that play a significant role in your stress response and whether you feel on edge or relaxed.

One of the keys to getting your hormones under control is to properly support your digestive health. In addition to eating the proper diet and drinking enough water, it's beneficial to:

- Eat probiotic-rich foods, like sauerkraut, kimchi, kefir, and kombucha.
- Take a high-quality probiotic.
- Eat prebiotic-rich foods, like chicory root, dandelion greens, Jerusalem artichoke, garlic, onions, leeks, and green bananas.
- Take prebiotics.
- Drink bone broth.
- Take collagen.

- Consider other gut-supporting supplements, like L-glutamine, bovine colostrum, and zinc carnosine.
- Get quality sleep.

Reducing your stress levels also has a huge effect on your gut health, so as you prioritize your stress management and reverse burnout, you'll also notice natural improvements in your digestion and your overall health.

Ditch Endocrine Disruptors

Endocrine disruptors, also called endocrine-disrupting compounds, or EDCs, are chemicals that interfere with normal hormone signaling. These types of chemicals can affect several hormonal systems in your body and negatively affect:

- Reproduction
- Thyroid function
- Nervous system function
- Digestion
- Blood sugar and insulin regulation

Because your hormonal systems are so sensitive, and very small fluctuations in hormone levels are enough to trigger changes in your body, even low doses of EDCs can lead to health problems.

Some common endocrine disruptors include:

- Bisphenol A (or BPA)—used to make plastic bottles and storage containers.
- Perchlorate—commonly found in drinking water.
- Perfluoroalkyl and polyfluoroalkyl substances (PFAS)—used to make many nonstick pans.
- Phthalates—used to make plastics more flexible, also found in cosmetic products, children's toys, and some food packaging.
- Polybrominated diphenyl ethers (PBDEs)—used to make flame retardants for furniture, mattresses, and carpets.
- Triclosan—found in hand sanitizer and some personal care products, like liquid body wash. Also registered with the FDA as a pesticide.

Go Organic

Some pesticides applied to conventional foods are known endocrine disruptors. When you eat these pesticide-treated foods, these chemicals can get into your bloodstream and affect your hormone balance. Because hormones are so sensitive, sometimes it takes only a small amount to throw things off-balance.

As a way to avoid hormone disruption, try to eat organic food as much as you can afford to. If you have a tight food budget, prioritize which foods and vegetables to buy organic by looking at the Environmental Working Group's Dirty Dozen and Clean Fifteen lists. The Dirty Dozen are the foods that have the most pesticide residue, while the Clean Fifteen are the foods with the least. If you have to pick and choose which produce to buy organic, prioritize the Dirty Dozen.

The lists change slightly each year, but as of 2020, the Dirty Dozen, which is actually thirteen foods, consists of:

- Strawberries
- Spinach
- Kale
- Nectarines
- Apples
- Grapes
- Peaches
- Cherries
- Pears
- Tomatoes
- Celery
- Potatoes
- Hot peppers

You can stay up-to-date on the most current Dirty Dozen and Clean Fifteen lists by checking the Environmental Working Group's website at www.ewg.org. Think about how you prepare your food too. If you're using a nonstick pan, especially one that has scratches in the coating, you're likely contaminating your food with endocrine disruptors during cooking. Try to stick to stainless-steel, cast-iron, and/or ceramic cookware.

Choose Nontoxic Beauty Products

You may not realize that the beauty products you're using—lotions, makeup, shampoo, body wash, deodorant, and so on—can affect the way that you feel, but they can play an important role in your health. Your skin is actually an organ, the biggest organ you have, and the things that you put on it get absorbed directly into the bloodstream. Certain areas, like your scalp, underarms, and groin area, are especially absorbent; depending on the product, these areas can take in almost 100 percent of whatever you put on them. That's why it's important to be as diligent about what you're putting on your body as you are about what you're eating.

The majority of beauty and skincare products on the shelves contain endocrine disruptors, cancer-causing chemicals, allergens, and/or general irritants.

To protect yourself, read ingredient labels on your beauty and skincare items and avoid harmful ingredients like:

- Fragrance/parfum
- Parabens
- Sulfates
- Phenoxyethanol (this one is common in "natural" products)
- Aluminum
- DEA (diethanolamine), MEA (monoethanolamine), and TEA (triethanolamine)
- PEG (polyethylene glycol)
- PG (propylene glycol) and butylene glycol
- Mineral oil
- SLS (sodium lauryl sulfate) and SLES (sodium laureth sulfate)
- Anything that ends in -siloxane or -methicone
- Triclosan

This isn't an exhaustive list, but it's a good start.

Swap Out Your Cleaning Supplies

Many conventional cleaning products contain potentially harmful, toxic chemicals that have been linked to infertility, increased risk of birth defects, allergies, asthma, and even cancer. A lot of these chemicals are also endocrine disruptors and can interfere with your hormonal balance and thyroid function.

When you breathe these chemicals in, they travel right into your bloodstream, where they can wreak havoc on your body without you even realizing it. These chemicals are also absorbed through your skin, like when you touch a disinfectant wipe to clean the counter.

Here are some of the most common endocrine disruptors that can be found in household cleaning products:

- Cyclosiloxanes (hexamethylcyclotrisiloxane, dodecamethylcyclohexasiloxane)
- Glycol ethers (e.g., 2-butoxyethanol, 2,[2-methoxyethoxy]ethanol)
- Phthalates (e.g., DEHP, DEP, DBP)
- Parabens (e.g., methylparaben, propylparaben)
- Alkylphenols (e.g., nonylphenols, octylphenols)
- Ethanolamides (e.g., monoethanolamine, diethanolamine)
- Triclosan

Other toxic chemicals often found in household cleaners include:

- Diethylene glycol monomethyl ether
- Borax and boric acid
- 1,4-Dioxane
- Formaldehyde (sometimes called formalin)

- Bleach (sodium hypochlorite)
- Ammonia (ammonium hydroxide)
- Quaternary ammonium compounds (e.g., benzalkonium chloride)
- Ethanolamines (mono-, di-, and triethanolamine)
- Sulfuric acid
- Perchloroethylene

Household cleaning supplies are not the only offenders: Be sure to read the ingredients list for things like laundry detergents, dryer sheets, candles, and scented plug-ins too. When you're trying to balance your hormones and manage your stress levels, it's important to clean up the environment and the air around you.

Do your best to switch to natural cleaning products. If you do use toxic cleaners, make sure you're always working in a well-ventilated area. Wear gloves, open windows and doors, and step outside for some fresh air as often as you can.

Get Rid of Plastic

A 2011 study published in *Environmental Health Perspectives* found that most commercial plastics, even those labeled as BPA-free, release chemicals that can mimic the actions of estrogen in your body. Exposing yourself to these kinds of plastics can significantly affect your hormone levels—and you might not even realize it!

Nowadays, it's impossible to avoid plastic completely, but there are ways you can reduce your plastic use:

- Replace plastic food containers with glass or stainless-steel options. If you do use plastic containers, avoid storing acidic or fatty foods in them and never put them in the microwave.
- Ditch plastic storage bags and use beeswax cloth in place of cling wrap.
- Choose beauty products that come in glass bottles or jars instead of plastic.
- When you get takeout, use real utensils instead of the plastic ones it comes with.

These may seem like insignificant changes, but they can add up. You probably don't realize how much plastic you're using—and the potential endocrine-disrupting chemicals you're exposed to—until you start paying attention to it.

Stay Active

Some studies link regular exercise to a lower risk of developing breast cancer. Why is that? It has to do with hormones. A sedentary life not only leads to weight gain; it can also increase your estrogen levels, which can increase your risk of hormone-related cancers, like breast cancer. On the other hand, exercise and staying active in general helps balance estrogen and can reduce your risk of serious health problems. Exercise also decreases your cortisol levels and makes your body physically stronger and more resilient to stress. When you feel physically stronger, you feel mentally stronger too.

Setting aside scheduled time to exercise, like thirty to sixty minutes a day, is great, but it's also a good idea to be as active as possible during the rest of the day. Take the stairs instead of the elevator. If you spend the day working at a desk, get up and walk around for a little bit every hour. Take walks after dinner. Do whatever you can to keep your body moving.

Keep in mind, though, that intense exercise can actually negatively affect your adrenal glands and cortisol levels. If you're dealing with stress overload or burnout, limit your activity to low or moderate intensity and don't push yourself too hard. The goal should be to simply move your body, not necessarily to burn as many calories as possible or drench yourself in sweat.

Choose Your Foods Wisely

Everything that goes into your mouth gets broken down into smaller components so that your body can use it to make new cells and structures. If you're relying on processed and sugary foods to get you through the day, your body will not be in peak form and you're probably going to be a stressed-out, anxious mess.

On the other hand, if you're paying attention to what you're eating and making healthy choices most of the time, your body will respond appropriately. Getting all of the necessary nutrients makes you more resilient to stress and gives you the mental energy you need to make the lifestyle changes necessary to tackle stress.

That doesn't mean you can't have processed foods or a sugary treat every now and then, but the focus of your diet should be on optimizing nutrient intake. What this looks like exactly depends on your specific dietary needs and goals. This usually will mean:

- Buying organic whenever possible
- Choosing grass-fed meats and pasture-raised poultry
- Getting pasture-raised eggs (and eating the yolks!)
- Choosing grass-fed dairy
- Going for wild-caught fish over farm-raised
- Including plenty of omega-3-rich seafood
- Eating lots of fruits and vegetables
- Avoiding gluten as much as possible
- Varying your food choices and eating lots of different colors
- Choosing sprouted grains
- Avoiding sugar and processed foods

Ditch the Low-Fat Mentality

Dietary fat has been a major source of contention for decades. But fat is nothing to fear. In fact, many of the health problems that are blamed on fat are actually sugar's fault.

Healthy fats not only provide you with important nutrients, like vitamins A, D, E, and K, but dietary fats are also essential to proper hormonal balance, ovulation, and fertility. And this doesn't only apply to unsaturated fats; there are plenty of saturated fats, like those that come from grass-fed meats and coconut oil, that are good for you too. Examples of healthy fats are:

- Grass-fed beef
- Pasture-raised chicken
- Grass-fed butter
- Avocados/avocado oil
- Ghee (clarified butter)
- Chia and hempseeds
- Flaxseeds
- Olives/olive oil
- Coconut/coconut oil
- Eggs

Pay attention to omega-3 fatty acids too. Your body uses omega-3s to make certain hormones, so if you don't get enough, it can lead to hormonal imbalances and health problems. Adequate omega-3 intake has even been associated with increased fertility and fetal health.

To ensure that you're getting enough healthy omega-3s:

- *Eat fatty fish.* Make salmon, anchovies, mackerel, sardines, or tuna your main protein source at least twice a week.
- *Eat nuts and seeds.* Walnuts and flaxseeds are excellent high-omega-3 options.
- *Take a high-quality fish oil supplement.* The extra-virgin cod liver oil from Rosita is a great option.

Get Connected

In today's world, it's easy to become socially isolated. You have social media to give you the illusion of connection, but, in reality, people are more disconnected than ever and it's doing a number on stress levels.

Social isolation and loneliness increase cortisol levels. The same is true of tense, unsupportive relationships—either romantic or platonic. Social isolation can also reduce enzymes that make GABA, a neurotransmitter that helps you relax and reduce anxiety. In one animal study published in the *Proceedings of the National Academy of Sciences of the United States of America*, researchers found that loneliness can reduce the enzymes that make GABA by as much as 50 percent!

On the other hand, close human bonds improve physical and mental health. And human touch—like a lingering hug or holding someone's hand—can lower cortisol while triggering the release of oxytocin, a hormone linked to relaxation, trust, and better mental health. Human touch also stimulates the vagus nerve, one of the major nerves that connects your brain to your body. When the vagus nerve is stimulated, it relaxes your nervous system and shuts down your stress response.

Regardless of whether you're busy with work, school, or kids, make time to see people in person, even if it's just to grab a quick coffee or tea or take a walk together. Give your friends hugs and cuddle with your significant other. Surround yourself with positive friends and family members who want to see you succeed with your goals and help you get there. Even better if you can find a family member or friend to start intermittent fasting with you so you can use each other as a source of support.

Ask for Help

Sometimes life's stressors are just too much to handle on your own, and when that happens, all of the do-it-yourself stress reduction and self-care techniques in the world might not be enough to help. In this case, you may benefit from seeing a therapist or someone who is properly trained in effective techniques like biofeedback and cognitive behavioral therapy.

There's no shame in talking with a professional who can help you navigate through your life stress in an unbiased way. If you've tried therapy in the past and didn't have a good experience with it, give it another try. Sometimes you have to go through several therapists before you find one that you really jibe with.

It's also beneficial to ask for help in your daily and home life. According to Linda Babcock, head of the Social and Decision Sciences Department at James M. Walton and founder of the Program for Research and Outreach on Gender Equity in Society (PROGRESS), many women don't ask for help at home. And taking on all of the burden of domestic duties can create stress that leads to resentment and burnout. If you feel like you're juggling too much, ask for help from your partner or your children. If you live alone, call your parents or a friend and ask if they can come over and help you or watch the kids while you take a break. Asking for help is not a sign of weakness or failure. You don't always need to do it all.

4

Best Fasting Approaches for Women

Once you've gotten your stress under control and your hormones balanced, it's time for the main event: easing into fasting! This chapter will guide you through the whole process, from deciding when you're ready to start fasting to choosing the best fasting approach for you. Remember: As a woman, it's always best to go slowly and see how you feel and then make adjustments from there.

Your goal should be to find the shortest fast that will give you positive results, instead of trying to fast for as long as you can. Don't try to power through a twenty-four-hour fast just so you can say you did it. You want to figure out what works for you without throwing off your hormones, and this chapter can help you get there.

Decide When You're Ready to Start Fasting

One of the most important steps to intermittent fasting is deciding when you're ready—or more accurately, when your body is ready—to start fasting. This is a non-negotiable part of the process that will ultimately determine whether or not you feel good when you start fasting. If you begin too soon, you can activate a negative hormone cascade that will only set you back.

That doesn't mean you have to be in perfect, shining health to start fasting. After all, you may be interested in fasting in the first place to correct some weight issues or health problems that you're dealing with. But you do have to make sure you have a handle on your stress levels, your adrenal glands are in decent shape, and you're not totally overwhelmed by life in general.

Some signs that you're ready to start fasting are:

- You don't feel completely overwhelmed by stress.
- You have enough energy to get through the day.
- You feel rested (or at least somewhat rested) when you wake up in the morning.
- Exercise makes you feel tired but energized, instead of completely drained.
- You're able to feel relaxed, rather than completely wound up all the time.

Again, you don't have to be full of energy, bouncing out of your bed at 6 a.m. when your alarm goes off to start fasting, but you should feel at least a little energized throughout the day and not like you're about to collapse under the weight of the world on your shoulders.

Ease Into Fasting Instead of Diving Right In

Once you decide that you're ready to start fasting, it's a good idea to ease into it instead of diving right in. Figuring out some small, actionable steps that you can take, and building on these steps over time, can help keep you from getting overwhelmed and make it easier to stick to intermittent fasting for the long term.

The best way to ease in depends on what your eating habits look like now. For example, if you're used to eating five or six small meals or three large meals and several snacks throughout the day, it might take longer to transition to a regular fasting schedule than it would for someone who eats only three meals with no snacks in between. In the beginning stages, forget following a specific fasting protocol and, instead, make small changes that will make your final transition easier.

If you're someone who eats a lot of snacks, make it your first goal to stick to meals only. Once you've nailed that goal, move on to skipping breakfast. When that becomes easy, start eating your dinner earlier, by a half hour or an hour at a time. Making small goals, and hitting them, will help your body adjust so it's not in total shock when you start fasting.

Crescendo Fasting

If you're brand-new to fasting—or you've tried other forms of fasting with negative results—it's a good idea to start with crescendo fasting. The word *crescendo* means "a gradual increase in intensity," and this is exactly how it works with crescendo fasting. With this form of intermittent fasting, you fast for twelve to fourteen hours a few days per week, rather than for sixteen hours every day. It's best to make these fasting days nonconsecutive, like Monday, Wednesday, and Friday, for example. The major point of crescendo fasting is to ease in slowly to avoid shocking the body too much at once so that your hormones don't react negatively.

If you feel good after crescendo fasting for a couple of weeks, you can add another day each week and see how your body reacts. If you still feel good, you can add more days until you reach your ultimate fasting goals. If you start with crescendo fasting and feel great, but you notice negative effects when you add longer or more frequent periods of fasting, you can always scale back and stay with a crescendo fasting schedule.

While sixteen-hour daily fasts are a common strategy, there's no one size fits all when it comes to intermittent fasting or some elusive goal that you have to meet to make sure you're doing it "right." Stick with what feels good for you.

Time-Restricted Fasting

Time-restricted fasting is the most popular and well-known form of intermittent fasting. With time-restricted fasting, you choose a specific eating window and a specific fasting window and stick to it every day. For example, you may choose to eat between the hours of 8 a.m. and 6 p.m. and then fast for the remaining time, between 6 p.m. and 8 a.m.

One of the reasons that time-restricted fasting is so popular is because it's easy to work it into your personal schedule. If you go to bed early and wake up early, you can make your eating window earlier in the day, but if you like to stay up a little later, you can push your eating window off to 8 p.m. Most of the fasting time occurs overnight and sleeping through eight hours of your fast is a lot easier than being awake for the entire duration.

While there are no specific rules about how long your fasting window should be during time-restricted fasting, it's usually between fourteen and sixteen hours. However, most experts recommend that women stick to the fourteen-hour fasting window to reduce the risk of any potential hormonal disruptions.

If you're worried you won't get the full benefit from fasting for only fourteen hours instead of sixteen, don't be. In a study published in *Cell Metabolism* in 2019, researchers found that fasting for fourteen hours could lead to:

- Weight loss
- Reduced waist circumference
- Decreased body fat and visceral fat
- Lowered blood pressure

- Decreased cholesterol and triglycerides

What's arguably most impressive is that the participants in this study all had metabolic syndrome, which can often make weight loss even harder, and they didn't change anything else about their diet. All they did was incorporate time-restricted fasting for twelve weeks.

The 16/8 (Leangains) Method

The 16/8 method, also referred to as the Leangains protocol, is a type of time-restricted fasting. When following the 16/8 method, you design your day around a sixteen-hour fasting window and an eight-hour feeding window. That means that every day you'll eat all of your meals within a consecutive eight-hour time frame and then you'll go the remaining sixteen hours without eating.

One of the benefits to this method is that, other than the length of the fasting and feeding windows, there are no specific timing rules; you can adjust the schedule to whatever works for you. For example, you can choose to eat between 10 a.m. and 6 p.m. and then fast between 6 p.m. and 10 a.m. If that doesn't suit you, you can make your eating window between noon and 8 p.m. and your fasting window between 8 p.m. and noon.

The one guideline to follow with the 16/8 method is to keep your schedule consistent each day. According to Martin Berkhan, a nutritional expert, personal trainer, and creator of this form of fasting, following the same schedule every day helps balance your hormones and give you the best results. On the other hand, if you're inconsistent with your schedule, it can throw off your hormones, leading to increased hunger and making it harder to stick to the program.

When following the 16/8 method, you can eat breakfast, lunch, and dinner and even a snack, as long as you're fitting it all into your eight-hour eating window.

Alternate-Day Fasting

Alternate-day fasting involves fasting every other day and then eating whatever you want on the other days, called "feast days." The most common way to do alternate-day fasting is by limiting your calorie intake to 25 percent of your needs on fasting days and then eating 125 percent of your calorie needs on feast days. For example, if you need 2,000 calories per day to sustain your energy, then you would eat 500 calories on Tuesday, Thursday, and Saturday and 2,500 calories on Monday, Wednesday, Friday, and Sunday.

Unlike with time-restricted feeding, alternate-day fasting has no rules about meal timing on your fasting days. You can eat your calories at breakfast, lunch, or dinner or have a couple smaller meals throughout the day. The choice is yours.

And research shows that whatever choice you make, you'll see benefits. In a small study published in *Obesity* in 2014, researchers put alternate-day fasters into three groups: lunch, dinner, and small meals. The lunch group ate all of their calories at lunch, the dinner group ate all of their calories at dinner, and the small meals group spread out their food intake throughout the day. At the end of the eight-week trial period, all participants experienced similar weight loss and overall improvements in their health.

If you don't have weight to lose, but want to reap some of the other benefits of fasting, other studies show that alternate-day fasting can reduce inflammation and lower LDL cholesterol. Alternate-day fasting can also improve your body composition by reducing body fat percentage and helping you retain lean body mass.

The 5:2 Method

The 5:2 method, also called the fast diet, is similar to alternate-day fasting, but instead of fasting every other day, you fast on two nonconsecutive days of the week and eat normally on the other five days. Also similar to alternate-day fasting, this method has you eating about 500–600 calories on each of your fasting days.

With the 5:2 method, your week might look like this:

- Monday: eat normally
- Tuesday: eat normally
- Wednesday: fast (eat 500–600 calories)
- Thursday: eat normally
- Friday: eat normally
- Saturday: fast (eat 500–600 calories)
- Sunday: eat normally

Keep in mind that there's not a single answer to what constitutes "normal" eating. What's normal for you depends on several factors, like your height, weight, sex, activity level, and overall goals. For example, if you're trying to lose weight, your normal eating days will look a lot different compared to someone who's trying to gain weight. There are several free online calculators you can use that will tell you your ideal calorie and macronutrient ranges based on your personal details, your goals, and your dietary preferences. Just search "online calorie calculator" or "online macronutrient calculator."

What Is Your Circadian Rhythm?

Your circadian rhythm, also sometimes referred to as your sleep/wake cycle, is a twenty-four-hour internal "clock" that regulates sleepfulness and wakefulness—or how awake and/or tired you feel during the course of a day. It's controlled by your hypothalamus, an area in your brain that's sensitive to light. When your hypothalamus senses light, it tells your body that it's time to wake up. Conversely, when it gets dark, your hypothalamus sends signals out that it's time to go to sleep. But while light is a huge factor in your circadian rhythm, it's also regulated by your eating schedule.

At optimal function, cortisol rises in the morning, reaches its peak at around 7 a.m., and then steadily drops throughout the day, reaching its lowest point at bedtime, around 9 p.m. or 10 p.m. Melatonin does the opposite; it's lowest in the morning and then steadily rises as the day goes on. In theory, these synergistic hormones would have you feeling energized and ready to tackle the day in the morning, and then sleepy at night when the sun goes down and bedtime approaches.

While your circadian rhythm is highly involved in your sleep patterns, it actually affects a lot of other bodily functions too. In the short term, disruptions in your circadian rhythm can cause lack of energy, difficulty remembering things, and poor wound healing.

In the long term, having a circadian rhythm that is out of whack can lead to:

- Diabetes
- Obesity
- Anxiety and depression
- Heart disease
- Metabolic diseases
- Digestive complaints and/or diseases
- Skin issues, like acne

Circadian Rhythm Fasting

With circadian rhythm fasting, you time your meals with the rise and fall of the sun and the corresponding surges and dips in cortisol, which has an effect on your thyroid hormones and metabolism too. When cortisol levels in your blood are high in the early hours, your metabolism is ready to go and much of the food you eat is used as energy. But when your cortisol goes down later in the day, your metabolism slows down with it, making it more likely that the food you eat will be stored as fat.

Circadian rhythm fasting likely looks very similar to how you've been told you *should* be eating. With circadian rhythm fasting, you stop eating at 7 p.m. every night and fast overnight for twelve hours, before eating again at 7 a.m.

In addition to timing your meals, circadian rhythm fasting involves making sure you're on a normal sleep schedule, which means going to bed and waking up at the same time every day and trying to fall asleep before 11 p.m.

Even though your eating window is a bit larger with this type of fasting, it's a good idea to eat only two or three meals instead of eating a bunch of smaller meals or snacking throughout the day. Getting outside in the sun for a few minutes when you first wake up can also help activate your hypothalamus, reducing melatonin and resetting your internal clock. If you can't go outside right when you wake up, you can experience some of this benefit by opening the blinds or curtains first thing in the morning.

Circadian Rhythm Fasting and Your Hormones

Circadian rhythm fasting can help balance hormones and improve the way you metabolize food when you have normal daily fluctuations in cortisol levels and hormonal cycles. If your cortisol level gets too high—like in times of chronic stress—it can actually have a paradoxical effect where cortisol increases your body fat, especially in the belly area, instead of helping you use food for energy. That's another reason why it's important to get your stress levels under control before you start any kind of intermittent fasting regimen.

Circadian rhythm fasting also affects the way insulin works in your body. When you eat, especially a high-carbohydrate meal, your blood sugar rises and your pancreas releases insulin to bring it down. If insulin rises at odd times—like when you eat a meal or snack late at night—it can throw off your circadian rhythm and increase your risk for long-term health problems, like type 2 diabetes and heart disease.

Insulin also promotes the storage of body fat, especially if you eat too many carbohydrates or calories, so you don't want it to be high at night right before bed when you're not expending a lot of energy.

Spontaneous Fasting

As the name implies, spontaneous fasting involves skipping meals whenever the desire strikes. There's no advance planning; you simply don't eat when you're not hungry. For example, if you're not hungry when you wake up, you skip breakfast instead of forcing yourself to eat it just because it's been called "the most important meal of the day." Or if lunchtime arrives and you're still full from breakfast, skip lunch and eat your next meal at dinnertime.

Many have been sold the idea that it's necessary to eat three meals every day, but there's no real rhyme or reason to this recommendation in the modern day. Eating three meals a day actually started with European settlers to make eating around working hours easier; the habit eventually spread to the rest of the world. On the other hand, Native Americans listened to their bodies and ate whenever they felt hungry, instead of based on what a clock said.

Spontaneous fasting is a good way to get your feet wet and see how you like the idea of skipping meals before you fully commit to a specific schedule. However, there are no rules here either. If you start with spontaneous fasting and you really like it, you don't have to move on to any other forms. You can stick with it indefinitely.

Making healthy food choices is always important, but it's especially critical with spontaneous fasting. Since there's no real structure to the plan and you don't know when you might be skipping a meal, you want to make sure you're optimizing your nutrient intake during all the meals that you do eat.

Choosing the Best Plan for You

Once you've familiarized yourself with all of the recommended fasting approaches for women, it's time to pick the one that resonates with you. It's important to make sure that whatever fasting plan you choose fits into your schedule. If it doesn't work with your current work and home routine, it's highly unlikely that you'll be able to sustain it long term.

And here's the great news: You don't have to follow any of the plans *exactly*. Mix and match the things you like from different plans to create a schedule that truly works for you. There's a lot of flexibility to intermittent fasting, and as long as you're feeling great while you do it, you don't have to get caught up in the stress of trying to do it "perfectly." Rigid rules can create more stress rather than helping to get rid of it. You want to make sure you're enjoying what you're doing to some degree or you'll never be able to stick with it.

Figuring Out Your Fasting Schedule

Once you've determined which type of intermittent fasting you want to do, the next step is to figure out your fasting schedule and actually write it down. Seriously, don't skip this part. Research shows that writing down a schedule makes it more likely that you'll stick to it. And you'll get major bonus points if you can see your schedule every day. Hang a wall calendar in the kitchen or write your weekly or monthly schedules out on a large dry-erase board that you can update in real time.

If you're doing time-restricted fasting, you'll want to figure out what time you'll stop eating, how long your fasting window will last, and when you'll start eating again. For example, if you decide you want to stop eating by 7 p.m. and your fasting window will last fourteen hours, your schedule will look like this:

- **Feeding window:** 9 a.m. to 7 p.m. (you'll eat all of your meals within this time frame)
- **Fasting window:** 7 p.m. to 9 a.m. (you'll stop eating your dinner by 7 p.m. every night and won't eat again until 9 a.m. the next morning)

Since time-restricted fasting is typically done every day of the week, once you figure out these numbers, you'll just stick to the same plan as long as you're feeling good and seeing benefits.

If you're doing a different fasting schedule, like alternate-day fasting or 5:2, all you need to do is figure out which days are going to be your eating days and which days will be your fasting days. For example, for alternate-day fasting you may decide to fast on Tuesdays, Thursdays, and Saturdays, and eat normally on the remaining days.

Sticking to Your Fasting Schedule

Once you've figured out a fasting schedule that works for you, do your best to stick to that schedule every week, even on the weekends when your schedule might be a little more relaxed. When you keep to the same schedule, it not only gives your body a chance to adapt and get used to fasting, but it also helps balance your hormones and make it more likely that you'll have a positive experience.

Of course, there are going to be times when something comes up, like a party or an early brunch with friends. When these things happen and you want to indulge, by all means, go for it, even if these events fall on your scheduled fasting days. A few off-schedule days here and there aren't going to totally mess up your progress, and having fun and going out is an important part of making sure you don't get too stressed.

The overall message here is to make sure you're sticking to the same fasting schedule *most* of the time, but don't beat yourself up if it's not all of the time.

Intermittent Fasting Schedules to Avoid

There are several different types of intermittent fasting schedules that can work for women, but there are others that can put more strain on the hormones and make it more likely that you'll experience negative results, especially if you have a lot of bad stress in your life. The following intermittent fasting practices are generally not recommended for women, unless you're experienced with fasting and you know that your body responds positively.

- **Eat Stop Eat:** Alternates one to two twenty-four-hour fasts each week with five to six normal eating days. For example, you would completely fast on Monday and Friday, but eat your normal diet, without any food or calorie restrictions, on the other days.
- **The Warrior Diet:** Divides the day into a twenty-hour undereating phase and a four-hour overeating phase. During the day, you can eat light snacks, like berries, yogurt, and whey protein, and drink vegetable juices, coffee, tea, and water. However, you're advised to eat only one large meal at night.
- **Extended Fasting:** Involves fasting for more than twenty-four hours, often a week or more, and drinking only water. These types of fasts should be done only in a medical setting. You should never do an extended fast without the recommendation and close supervision of a medical professional who is also trained in proper refeeding protocols.

Who Shouldn't Fast at All

Once stress levels are under control, intermittent fasting is an appropriate strategy for most healthy women. However, there are certain categories of women who should not fast at all. You should completely avoid intermittent fasting if you are:

- Pregnant or breastfeeding
- Severely underweight
- Malnourished or have significant nutrient deficiencies
- Under eighteen years of age
- Experiencing cortisol dysregulation and/or stress overload

You should speak to your doctor or a qualified nutritionist who's familiar with your personal medical history before trying fasting if you:

- Are taking any medications
- Have a history of disordered eating
- Have diabetes (type 1 or type 2)

When you have diabetes, your body has a harder time regulating blood glucose and insulin levels. This can make fasting a challenge, since, physiologically, your body doesn't respond as it should. However, research shows that fasting may help improve insulin sensitivity, reverse insulin resistance, and return fasting blood glucose levels to normal in people with type 2 diabetes. The biggest concern with fasting when you have diabetes is the potential for hypoglycemia, or low blood sugar, but this is more common in type 1 diabetes than type 2 diabetes. If you have type 2 diabetes and want to see if fasting can help, talk to your doctor before starting and make sure you're closely monitoring your blood sugar levels.

Fasting and Eating Disorder Recovery

There's no evidence that fasting can trigger disordered eating in women without a history of eating disorders. But if you're currently in recovery from an eating disorder, or you suspect that you may have an eating disorder, it's best to avoid any eating style that restricts food in any way.

Some signs of disordered eating include:

- Obsessing about food or weight
- Talking incessantly about food, weight, or your diet
- Negative body image or obsession with body image
- Isolating yourself from others so you don't have to eat
- Avoiding social events for food-related reasons
- Anxiety around eating food

If you're experiencing any of these signs, intermittent fasting could be doing more harm than good. The goal is to make it a positive experience in your life, not one that you obsess over. If you recognize any disordered eating patterns in yourself, seek out advice and guidance from a qualified health team that includes a psychologist and a nutritionist qualified in navigating eating disorders.

Getting Enough Calories

It's important to stress the fact that intermittent fasting is not necessarily meant to be a calorie-restricted plan. You may eat fewer calories than you were eating before—especially if you're coming from a standard American diet where you didn't pay much attention to portion sizes—but the goal isn't to restrict your calories in the same way that low-calorie diets do.

You might think that restricting your calories is a good way to lose weight fast, but calorie restriction can have detrimental effects, especially on women. There's plenty of research that shows:

- Following a low-calorie diet can reduce your basal metabolic rate (or the amount of calories you burn doing nothing) by as much as 23 percent. This can continue for years, even after you start eating normally again.
- Calorie restriction can cause muscle loss (fasting can actually increase lean muscle mass).
- Eating 22–42 percent fewer calories than needed to maintain normal weight can negatively affect fertility and reproductive function in women.
- Calorie restriction can cause reductions in testosterone and estrogen, which can reduce bone formation and weaken your bones.

It's also harder to get all of the nutrients you need when you're not eating enough calories, since fewer calories means less food overall. When you're intermittent fasting, you don't want to focus on getting fewer calories; you actually want to focus on getting only nutrient-dense calories—and making sure you're getting enough of them.

Figuring Out Your Calorie Needs

The amount of calories you need is based on two factors: resting energy expenditure (REE) and nonresting energy expenditure (NREE). Your REE represents the calories you burn at rest, or while you're sitting and doing nothing. Your NREE represents the calories you burn during physical activity, like when you're exercising. When you add these two numbers together, it gives you your total daily energy expenditure (TDEE).

That may seem complicated, but there are lots of free online calculators that will do the math for you. All you have to do is search for "online calorie calculator" and take your pick.

If you don't want to use an online calculator, you can plug your own information into what's called the Mifflin-St. Jeor equation. For women, it looks like this:

$$10 \times \text{weight (kg)} + 6.25 \times \text{height (cm)} - 5 \times \text{age (y)} - 161$$

If you're a thirty-three-year-old, 150-pound, 5'6" woman and you plug your stats into the equation, you get an REE of 1,403.

Once you have your REE, the next step is to determine your TDEE based on how much you exercise. To do this, all you have to do is multiply the number you get (1,403 in this example) by one of the following activity factors:

- **Sedentary:** 1.2 (light to no exercise)
- **Lightly active:** 1.375 (light exercise less than three days per week)
- **Moderately active:** 1.55 (moderate exercise most days of the week)
- **Very active:** 1.725 (moderate to intense exercise every day)
- **Extremely active:** 1.9 (strenuous exercise two or more times per day)

If you're lightly active, then based on the previous example, your TDEE would be 1,929 (which means your NREE is 526). To simplify things, you can round this number to 1,900. The TDEE represents how many calories you need each day to maintain your current weight.

Do You Have to Count Calories?

It's not really necessary to count calories if you're following a properly designed, nutrient-dense intermittent fasting plan. But in the initial stages, figuring out your calorie needs and then logging your food for a few weeks can help give you a general picture of how much food you're eating. Once you have a feel for the volume of food you should be eating, you don't have to keep going with the calorie counting if it's causing you too much stress.

The goal isn't to make sure you're sticking to an exact number—it's to make sure you're eating enough calories so you don't experience any of the negative health effects of excessive calorie restriction. It's also to give you a general sense of the volume of food you can eat while staying within your calorie goals.

If you've never counted calories before, you may be surprised by how much food you can eat for 1,900 calories when you're choosing nutrient-dense whole foods and lots of vegetables. Some women actually feel like they're eating too much, especially if they're used to a lifetime of calorie restriction.

The aim with intermittent fasting isn't to deny your body of foods; it's to delay the timing of that food.

Getting Enough Micronutrients

In addition to getting enough calories, you want to make sure you're getting plenty of micronutrients—or vitamins and minerals—when intermittent fasting. You often see a lot of focus on the macronutrients (carbohydrates, protein, and fat), but micronutrients are a huge underlying factor in whether you feel good and remain healthy or not.

If you're not getting enough micronutrients, it can lead to vitamin and mineral deficiencies that can potentially cause numerous negative symptoms and health problems. Some signs of a micronutrient deficiency include:

- Hair loss
- Restless leg syndrome
- Brittle nails
- Dry, cracked skin around the mouth
- Numbness and tingling in the extremities
- Numbness and tingling on your tongue
- Memory problems
- Confusion
- Dizziness
- Muscle aches and pains
- Anxiety
- Fatigue and weakness

Specific deficiencies, like vitamin B_{12} deficiency, can even lead to permanent nerve damage if they're not caught and corrected early enough.

This is why it's important to optimize your micronutrient intake each time you eat, especially since you'll be eating less often when intermittent fasting. To ensure that you're getting plenty of vitamins and minerals:

- Eat only whole, unprocessed foods.
- Include a wide variety of foods in your diet, instead of eating the same things over and over.
- Try to eat two or three colors at every meal, for example broccoli   . (green), tomatoes (red), and sweet potatoes (orange).
- Eat at least five servings of vegetables every day.

Determining the Right Diet for You

Although the term *diet* is most often connected to some type of food restriction or low-calorie program, the true definition of the word is the type of food that you habitually eat. And that's the way you should interpret it in this case.

You don't have to throw a label on the foods you're eating or follow any specific dietary dogma at all. The most important thing is to make sure you're getting plenty of nutrient-dense whole foods and optimizing your micronutrients at every meal. It's also important that you feel good with the food you're eating.

Many women decide to pair intermittent fasting with a low-carb or keto diet since fasting and keto both force your body to use up glucose and stored glycogen and start burning body fat, but that certainly isn't a requirement. You also don't have to follow a certain dietary plan exactly as written. For example, if you're drawn to a Paleo diet, but you love rice and you find that your body does well with it, you can add it in. The key is to make sure you're at your best and be honest with yourself about how certain foods make you feel. Design your diet around the foods that make you feel good and get rid of the ones that don't.

The Best Way to Break Your Fast

No matter which diet plan you choose to follow, it's best to break your fast with a low-glycemic meal that contains plenty of high-quality protein and some healthy fats. This helps fill you up quickly, while also keeping your blood sugar stable so you feel satisfied for longer. Conversely, you want to avoid sugary or carbohydrate-heavy foods for your first meal of the day. These types of foods spike your blood sugar and can cause a blood sugar roller coaster that also raises your insulin levels, leaving you feeling hungry and cranky.

It's also a good idea to pay attention to your portion sizes. Even if you feel really hungry when you're first starting out with fasting, stick to small meals or snacks when it's time to eat your first meal of the day. Eating too much at once can be hard on your digestive system and may cause gas, bloating, and general feelings of sluggishness and heaviness.

Some excellent choices for your first meal of the day are:

- Eggs
- Chicken
- Cooked vegetables
- Leafy greens
- Healthy fats (like grass-fed butter, olive oil, coconut oil, and avocado)
- Nut butters
- A small handful of berries
- Fermented foods (like plain yogurt or kefir, sauerkraut, and kimchi)
- Bone broth or soups

Taking Your Body Measurements

Many women rely on the scale to tell them whether or not they're making progress, but the scale isn't a good representation of all of the changes in your body composition that happen when you make intermittent fasting a regular part of your lifestyle. If weight loss is one of your major goals (and even if it isn't), make sure you take measurements before you add intermittent fasting into your lifestyle.

Measurements give you a much better picture of how well you're progressing because as you turn fat into lean muscle mass, you can lose inches and drop pant sizes without seeing significant dips in the numbers on the scale.

When taking your measurements, make sure you're wearing tight-fitting clothing or no clothing at all. If you choose to measure yourself clothed, try to wear the same clothes every time, unless they become really loose and baggy (and if you have some weight to lose, there's a good chance they will).

Next, grab a flexible measuring tape, a piece of paper, and a pen, and write down all of these values (you can also record them in a note on your smartphone):

- **Bust/Chest:** Measure around the chest, directly across your nipple line.
- **Waist:** Measure across your belly button.
- **Hips:** Place tape measure around the widest part of your hips.
- **Thighs:** Measure around the largest part of each thigh.
- **Arms:** Measure around the largest part of each upper arm.

Take your measurements every four weeks and be patient as you go. Small changes are still changes, and over time they all add up.

Is Fasting Working for You?

You can look at all the science and read all the theories in the world, but ultimately, whether or not intermittent fasting is working for you comes down to how your body is reacting. When you're starting a new intermittent fasting schedule, it's important to pay attention to both sudden and gradual changes in how you feel.

If your hunger and sugar cravings go away, you feel satisfied and full of energy, you're starting to slim down, and your skin is glowing, these are all excellent signs that your fasting program is working for you and you should stay the course.

However, if after a couple of weeks of fasting you feel run-down, cranky, and worse than ever, it might be time to go back to the drawing board. Some signs that your current intermittent fasting plan isn't working for you include:

- Mood swings
- Chronic fatigue
- Weight gain
- Decreased tolerance to stress
- Thinning hair or loss of hair
- Difficulty falling asleep or staying asleep
- Exhaustion after a workout or a harder time recovering from exercise
- Acne
- Dry skin
- Irregular menstrual cycles or complete cessation of your menstrual cycle
- Heart palpitations

- Decreased tolerance to cold temperatures or always feeling cold
- Digestive problems, like constipation, gas, and/or bloating
- Decreased sex drive
- Slow healing cuts
- Increased sickness, like always getting every bug going around

If you're experiencing any of these symptoms, it's a good idea to take a step back and continue working on stress management or change the type and length of fasting that you're doing. You may also benefit from addressing some other areas, like the type of exercise you're doing (and how often you're doing it), what kinds of foods you're eating, and whether or not you're drinking enough water.

5

Other Ways to Make Sure You Feel Good

Intermittent fasting is powerful on its own, but when you pay attention to other areas of your lifestyle, like what exactly you're eating, getting enough clean water, and following the right exercise schedule, you'll be blown away by how good you can feel. A lot of women don't realize it's possible to feel so good until they experience it for themselves.

This chapter goes beyond the principles of intermittent fasting and guides you through other changes you can make so that you can truly feel your best. If you want to get all you can out of an intermittent fasting lifestyle—or you started intermittent fasting and you're not seeing the results you hoped for—these tips can help you get there.

The Best Foods to Eat

One of the beautiful things about intermittent fasting is that you can see some pretty significant changes even if you don't completely overhaul your diet. That being said, focusing on getting most of your calories and nutrients from whole foods and limiting processed foods as much as possible will make a world of difference in how you feel.

You should design most of your meals around:

- Meat
- Poultry
- Seafood
- Vegetables

- Fruits
- Nuts and seeds
- Beans
- Healthy fats

And try to avoid:

- Packaged and heavily processed foods (chips, frozen dinners, crackers, canned soups)
- Refined carbohydrates (white pasta, white bread)
- Processed vegan foods/fake meats (Beyond Meat, Tofurkey, margarine, plant-based butter)
- Foods with added sugars (cookies, ice cream, cakes)
- Fast food
- Artificial sweeteners (Equal, Splenda, Sweet'N Low)
- Sugary drinks (soda, lemonade, sweet tea)

Minimally processed foods, like frozen or canned items without a lot of additives, are okay, but whenever you can prepare fresh foods, that's always best.

Choose High-Quality Foods

If you're not feeling your best, consider upgrading your food to as high a quality as your budget will allow. The best options are:

- **Grass-fed beef:** Contains up to five times more omega-3 fatty acids than conventional meat. It's as much as 500 percent higher in conjugated linoleic acid, a type of fat that acts as an antioxidant and has been shown to boost weight loss, reduce the risk of heart disease and type 2 diabetes, and help stop the growth of certain types of cancerous tumors.
- **Organic, pasture-raised chicken:** Higher in vitamins, minerals, and omega-3 fatty acids than conventional chicken.
- **Eggs from organic, pasture-raised hens:** Make sure you eat the yolks too. That's where most of the nutrients, like vitamins A, D, E, and K, B vitamins, omega-3 fatty acids, and calcium are found.
- **Wild-raised, smaller fish:** Wild fish are higher in omega-3 fatty acids than farm-raised fish. Small fish are less contaminated than larger fish, since they're lower in the food chain. The best choices are salmon, trout, sardines, mackerel, herring, oysters, and mussels.
- **Organic produce:** If your food budget is tight, prioritize the Dirty Dozen (see Chapter 3).
- **Unrefined, healthy oils:** Grass-fed butter and ghee, avocado oil, hemp oil, olive oil, and sesame oil are great choices.
- **Grass-fed, organic, and/or cultured dairy:** Grass-fed dairy has higher omega-3s and lower omega-6s than conventional dairy. Cultured dairy, like yogurt and kefir, contain probiotics that can help keep your gut healthy. Get plain versions instead of flavored ones, which usually contain a lot of sugar.

The Best Drink Choices

In a perfect world, water would be the only thing you drink, but nothing is perfect, so that's probably not going to happen. If you want to feel your best, stick to the following:

- Filtered water
- Organic coffee
- Tea (black, herbal, green)
- Matcha green tea
- Coconut water (check for added sugar)
- Almond milk
- Coconut milk
- Oat milk
- Hemp milk
- Flax milk

Plant-based milks, like almond, coconut, oat, hemp, and flax, can be a good option, especially if you're trying to avoid dairy, but when it comes to ingredients and quality, they run the gamut. For example, some almond milks, like Malk, are minimally processed and made with only water, almonds, and salt, while others are made with sugar and an artificial ingredient list that's a mile long, but hardly any almonds. Don't assume that a plant-based milk is healthy just because it isn't dairy. Read labels and choose unsweetened milks with a minimal number of ingredients.

You can also occasionally enjoy:

- Stevia-sweetened soda (not diet soda)
- Natural energy drinks, like Kill Cliff

These drinks don't have any added sugar, but they are sweetened with stevia and erythritol. While these sweeteners won't spike your blood sugar, they might make sugar cravings worse, especially if you're using them to try to combat a soda habit.

Get Enough Protein

It's important to get all of the nutrients you need on a regular basis, but protein is arguably *the* most important nutrient for a woman who is doing intermittent fasting. Getting enough protein will help prevent muscle loss, one of the main concerns centered on women and fasting. Protein can also help you lose weight and keeps you feeling full.

Some signs that you're not getting enough protein are:

- Feeling extremely fatigued or weak
- Feeling hungry most of the time
- Brittle hair and nails
- Dry, flaky skin
- Mood swings
- Getting sick often
- Feeling swollen or having swollen hands or feet

If you're dealing with these symptoms even after you've gotten your stress levels under control, it's possible that you need to eat more protein. Protein powders can help you up your protein intake, but it's best to meet your goals through whole foods since they provide lots of other nutrients too.

Aim for at least 0.36 grams of protein per pound of body weight. If you're 150 pounds, that means you need about 54 grams of protein per day. If you're 200 pounds, you need about 72 grams. For reference, 4 ounces of cooked chicken breast has about 34 grams of protein and ½ cup of cooked black beans has about 8 grams.

Eat More Fat

Protein gets a lot of credit for keeping you full, but fat, which has been vilified for a long time, deserves some credit too. Not only is fat one of the most satiating macronutrients; it also provides a sustained source of energy.

Research shows that when you eat foods that are rich in dietary fat, it stimulates receptors in your mouth and your small intestine that slow down the rate of digestion and release gut peptides—chemical messengers that regulate food intake—which can help keep you feeling full for a longer period of time. The only catch is that when you combine fat with sugar, it blunts the satiating effects. That's why it's so easy to overeat high-fat, high-carb foods, like ice cream and pizza, but it's unlikely that you'd overdo it on foods like avocado or olives.

Don't shy away from fat. You don't have to go crazy with it, but make sure it's part of all of your meals. Plain chicken and asparagus will keep you full for a little while, but if you toss the asparagus in some grass-fed butter, the satiating effects will last much longer.

Carbs and Your Cycle

If you're following a low-carb or keto diet along with your intermittent fasting protocol, you may benefit from increasing carbohydrates at the beginning of your cycle and right before your period starts. This approach, called carb cycling, can help keep hormones balanced and prevent your body from getting overwhelmed during times of stress (like your period).

Here's one of the best approaches to carb cycling around your period:

- Increase carbohydrates on days 3–5 of your cycle.
- Lower carbohydrates on days 6–21.
- Increase carbohydrates again on days 22–25.
- Decrease carbohydrates again until you get to day 3 of your next cycle.

During the times when you're upping your carb intake, your levels of the hormones estrogen and progesterone are fluctuating, and possibly making you crave high-carb and sweet foods.

However, if you decide to carb cycle, it's best to get your carbs from healthy nutrient-dense sources, like:

- Potatoes (sweet, purple, and white)
- Quinoa
- Buckwheat
- Bananas (and other fruits)
- Pumpkin
- Beans
- Chickpeas
- Beets
- Plain yogurt

It's okay to give in to a craving once in a while, but if you rely on sugary foods to increase your carb intake, you'll probably end up feeling worse in the long run.

Avoid Sugar As Much As Possible

Many of the health problems that have been blamed on fat are actually caused by sugar. Not only is sugar almost completely devoid of nutritional benefit, but it is also shown to cause chronic inflammation, mess up blood sugar and insulin levels, increase your risk of heart disease, and feed cancer cells. Sugar also makes it easier for you to gain weight and can increase anxiety and cause mood swings.

There are certain sugars, like honey and pure maple syrup, that are better for you than others, but the bottom line is that sugar is still sugar. While adding some honey to your tea or maple syrup to your coffee is okay (if you're drinking it during your feeding window), all sugar should be limited as much as possible if you want to feel your best.

That doesn't mean that you should replace sugar with artificial sweeteners. Studies show that people who regularly consume artificial sweeteners have increased risk of diabetes, metabolic syndrome, heart disease, cancer, and migraines. Artificial sweeteners can also throw off the balance of bacteria in your gut, causing digestive problems and widespread health issues. Another thing to consider is that when you give your body a sweet taste without any calories, it can make sugar cravings worse. So for many reasons it's best to limit sweeteners as much as you can.

If you do need something sweet, your best choices are:

- Erythritol
- Monk fruit
- Stevia (without added flavors or other artificial ingredients)
- Raw honey
- Pure maple syrup

The Problems with Gluten

Gluten is kind of a hot-button issue. Celiac disease, an autoimmune disorder in which eating gluten causes physical damage to the small intestine, has been widely recognized for years. On the other hand, non-celiac gluten sensitivity (or NCGS), an adverse reaction to eating gluten that doesn't cause damage to the intestine, has only recently become more acknowledged.

In the past, the medical community denied the existence of NCGS, or gluten intolerance as most people call it. But research now recognizes that gluten sensitivity is real and that people can have widespread inflammation and symptoms from eating gluten even if they don't have celiac disease.

Some of the most common symptoms of gluten sensitivity are:

- Gas and bloating
- Stomach pain
- Diarrhea or constipation
- Nausea
- Joint and/or muscle pain
- Numbness in the extremities
- Brain fog or fatigue
- Anxiety

This list isn't fully exhaustive, though. And Dr. Mark Hyman, a leading functional medicine physician, recommends avoiding gluten even if you aren't experiencing any noticeable symptoms. According to Dr. Hyman, gluten can trigger the release of an inflammatory protein called zonulin that creates openings in the gut, allowing food particles and other large proteins to get into the bloodstream, where they don't belong. This condition, called leaky gut, is an underlying cause of systemic inflammation and many chronic health problems.

Dr. Hyman also points out that many gluten-filled foods, like pastas, breads, and cereals, simply aren't that good for you, and when you base your diet around them, you push better, healthier foods off your plate.

Ditch Gluten

If gluten is still a part of your diet and you're feeling kind of "meh," it's probably a good idea to get rid of it, at least for a while, and see what happens. Try not to replace gluten-containing foods with gluten-free packaged foods, though. Even if these foods don't contain gluten, they're still processed and usually not very nutrient dense. It's best to ditch gluten and replace it with nutrient-dense whole foods and minimally processed gluten-free grains.

Some of the most common gluten-containing foods are:

- Breads and croutons
- Cereals
- Crackers
- Baked goods, like cakes, pies, and cookies
- Pastas
- Beer

Other, less obvious sources of gluten include:

- Frozen French fries
- Hot dogs
- Processed deli meats and cheeses
- Dressings and sauces
- Soups and soup mixes
- Gravy
- Snack foods, like potato chips and tortilla chips

Instead of eating these types of foods, build your diet around fruits, vegetables, protein, healthy fats and oils, nuts, and seeds.

Plan and Prep Your Meals in Advance

Sometimes just trying to figure out what and when to eat is enough to cause more stress than you'd like. That's why meal planning can be a great tool to help keep you feeling your best. It takes the guesswork out of eating, and you never have to worry about the specifics of your next healthy meal—two huge weights off your shoulders.

The first thing you need to do is design your meal plan by figuring out what you're going to eat and when. You can plan out a few days, a week, or even a full month. Find simple recipes or compile a list of your favorite go-to meals and write down which ones you're going to eat when. There are online meal planners and phone apps that you can use to make meal planning super easy, but if you prefer a good old-fashioned pen and paper, that's fine too!

Once you've figured out your meal schedule, the next step is meal prepping, which can include things like cooking meats and/or sides ahead of time and portioning foods out in storage containers. This certainly isn't a requirement, but research shows that people who prepare their meals in advance have an easier time sticking to their goals and have greater success than people who don't. Meal prepping can also save you money since you're not tempted to get takeout at the last minute and you're less likely to make impulse food purchases when you have your next meal ready to go.

Distract Yourself from Hunger

How many times have you thought you were hungry but you were really just bored? One minute you're relaxing on the couch, and the next minute you're searching through the pantry for something—anything—to snack on. Pretty soon, you're at the bottom of a bag of chips, or five Oreos deep, and you don't even know what happened.

When you get the urge to snack like this, find a way to distract yourself. One of the most effective things you can do is start an activity that involves your hands or lots of movement. Clean the house, respond to some emails, text a friend, or find a crafty hobby you like, such as drawing. If the temptation is really strong, go for a walk or run an errand—whatever gets you out of the house and away from the pantry.

It's also a good idea to avoid things that trigger emotional or psychological hunger. If seeing a bag of chips in the cabinet makes your mouth start watering immediately, keep chips out of the house or somewhere that's not so in your face.

Keep in mind that these suggestions are only to help you get through your fasting windows. If you feel hungry during your feeding window, eat!

Drink Lots of Water

To understand just how important water is, consider this: You could survive up to two months without food, but you would only last for a few days without water. Crazy, right? Drinking water not only makes sure everything in your body is working as it should—after all, you're made of about 60 percent water—it also:

- Keeps you full
- Helps you lose weight
- Allows you to shed water weight
- Prevents headaches and fatigue
- Gives you energy

But how much water do you need? The exact amount depends on different things, like your height and weight and the climate where you live, but here are some easy general water guidelines that you can follow:

- Drink at least half of your body weight in ounces every day. If you weigh 150 pounds, your baseline is 75 ounces of water.
- Add an extra 8 ounces of water for every caffeinated beverage you drink.
- Add an extra 8 ounces of water for every alcoholic beverage you drink.
- Add an extra 8 ounces of water for every fifteen minutes of exercise.

Make Sure Your Water Is Clean

After extensive testing, the Environmental Working Group (EWG) has identified around 278 contaminants in drinking water. Currently, under the Safe Drinking Water Act, the Environmental Protection Agency (EPA) regulates only ninety of those contaminants. That means that there are 188 possible known contaminants in your water that are going unmonitored and unregulated.

Contaminants fall into four major categories:

1. **Physical:** sediment from lakes and rivers
2. **Chemical:** pesticides, heavy metals, toxins, medications, bleach, and salts
3. **Biological:** bacteria, viruses, fungi, and parasites
4. **Radiological:** uranium, cesium, plutonium, and other unstable compounds

Tap water can also contain hormone-disrupting chemicals, including residues from birth control pills and other medications.

Because the definition of contaminant is so broad, the health effects from consuming contaminated water are also broad. Contaminated water can cause weight gain, nervous system disorders like multiple sclerosis, reproductive problems, digestive conditions, and even cancer.

Although your tap water is monitored, it's still possible that there are contaminants lurking in it. Often the contaminants are above the legal limits. If you search for "how many contaminants are in my water" online, you can find the EWG's tap water database to see how many contaminants have been detected in your water and how many exceed health guidelines. Even if the ninety regulated contaminants fall within legal limits, that doesn't necessarily mean they're safe to drink. Bottled water isn't the solution either, as it's even less regulated than tap water.

If you want to feel your best, it's important to make sure you're drinking clean filtered water. You can use refrigerator filters, like Brita or ZeroWater, but these still leave some contaminants behind. A whole-house filter that also filters your shower water is the gold standard, but if you don't have the budget for that, an under-sink filter is the next best option.

The Importance of Electrolytes

To stay properly hydrated, you need electrolytes, like sodium, potassium, and magnesium, in addition to water. Even if you're drinking enough water, low electrolytes can cause dizziness, fatigue, headaches, and confusion. If you're drinking too much water, it can actually dilute your electrolytes and force your body to expel more of them, so it's especially important to make sure things are balanced.

Most commercial electrolyte drinks are full of sugar, but Kill Cliff has a great line that's sweetened only with erythritol and stevia. You can stock up on those or you can make your own electrolyte drink by combining:

- Juice from ½ large lemon
- ⅛ teaspoon sea salt (Celtic or pink Himalayan)
- 8 ounces filtered water or coconut water
- 1 teaspoon raw honey

This is enough for one serving, but you can triple or quadruple the recipe and keep some in your refrigerator for whenever you're feeling a little low on energy and need a dose of electrolytes.

Make sure you're using Celtic sea salt or pink Himalayan salt. These are electrolyte-rich natural salts that come from dried salt water. Regular table salt has been filtered and processed and doesn't have the same minerals and electrolytes.

Spread Out Your Intake

In addition to getting enough water and electrolytes, it's helpful to spread out your water intake throughout the day. Your body can process only about 27–34 ounces of water per hour. If you drink more than that, it can actually work against you by diluting your electrolyte and sodium levels too much. If this happens, it can lead to a potentially dangerous condition called hyponatremia—the most common type of electrolyte imbalance.

Instead of chugging a bunch of water at once or waiting until the end of the day and then trying to catch up with your water needs, carry a water bottle around with you and sip from it often. Bone broth is also an excellent way to get the water and electrolytes you need. If you drink bone broth, just make sure to drink it only during your eating window since it has calories and amino acids that break your fast.

Exercise and Fasting

Like intermittent fasting, exercise can help stimulate autophagy, or cellular cleansing, in the body and in the brain. That's a major reason why, in addition to helping improve your heart health, exercise can also reduce your risk of cancer and neurodegenerative diseases, like Alzheimer's and Parkinson's, and improve brain function.

One study published in *Autophagy* found that autophagy increases significantly after jogging for thirty minutes on a treadmill and continues to increase for up to eighty minutes, when it begins to level out.

If you want to feel your best, make sure you're exercising regularly. While at least thirty minutes of structured exercise every day is best, even some low-intensity movement, like an after-dinner walk, will help improve the way you feel.

To Eat or Not to Eat Before a Workout

There's a lot of debate in the fitness world about whether it's better to exercise on an empty stomach (fasted state) or after you've eaten a proper meal (fed state). The answer to that really depends on the intensity of your workout. If you're doing high-intensity exercise or you're an endurance athlete, some experts would say that working out after you eat (but not too soon after) is probably a better idea. However, if you're doing lighter exercise, like walking or yoga, there are some benefits to exercising in a fasted state.

Exercising on an empty stomach can help improve levels of insulin and growth hormone. When you exercise in a fasted state, you're not only giving your body a longer break from releasing insulin into the blood; you're also using up any excess insulin that might still be hanging around from when you last ate. This helps improve insulin sensitivity and increases blood flow to your muscles, making it easier to burn fat and build muscle. As insulin sensitivity improves, production of growth hormone also goes up. Growth hormone helps your body burn fat, increase muscle tissue, and improve bone health.

But when it comes to fat loss, studies show no real difference. One study published in *Obesity* in 2013 found that high-intensity interval training could help get rid of excess fat, improve body composition, and improve the muscles' ability to burn fat, whether the women involved ate before exercise or not.

The bottom line is that the timing of your exercise—before your first meal or after—is your choice to be made depending on what your goals are.

Some General Exercise Guidelines

There are no hard-and-fast rules concerning exercising while fasting, but there are some general guidelines you can follow to ensure that you'll feel your best:

- **Do your cardio fasted.** Your body fat can power you through low- to moderate-intensity cardio. Even though there's conflicting information on whether or not fasted cardio helps you burn more fat, it doesn't hurt. If you want to do your cardio on an empty stomach, schedule it for first thing in the morning if you can.
- **Do low-intensity exercise whenever you want.** Lower-intensity exercises like yoga or tai chi don't require a lot of short bursts of energy, and they don't put the same stress on the body as higher-intensity workouts. If you're doing these types of workouts, you can do them whenever they best fit into your schedule.
- **Lift weights between or after meals.** Strength training requires a decent amount of energy, for you and your muscles, and eating before you lift weights makes it easier for you to build lean muscle. Schedule your lifting or strength training exercises during your eating window or right after it. For example, if your eating schedule is 11 a.m. to 8 p.m., you can do your lifting at lunchtime or right before dinner, or at 8:30 p.m. or 9 p.m.

How to Do High-Intensity Exercise

Low-intensity exercise is best for preventing stress overload when you're fasting, but that doesn't mean that you can't work some higher-intensity exercises, like high-intensity interval training (HIIT) or strength training, into your schedule too.

On the days when you want to do high-intensity exercise, time your training for about an hour after a meal. Although there are benefits of exercising in a fasted state, when you exercise in a fed state, the food in your system acts as a source of fuel. This gives you the energy you need to power through a more grueling workout. It can also help prevent muscle loss and keep your blood sugar levels from getting too low as you move.

A good way to gauge the intensity of your workout is by using what's called the talk test. If you're able to carry on a conversation fairly easily without getting out of breath while you work out, that exercise is considered low intensity. If you're only able to comfortably say a few words at a time, you're doing a high-intensity workout. If you can't talk at all during your workout without losing your breath, you might be exerting too much effort and it could be beneficial to scale back a little.

More Exercise Tips

Exercise and intermittent fasting go hand in hand. They both stimulate autophagy and keep you healthy and happy. But like intermittent fasting, exercise can turn into a bad stressor if you're not doing it correctly. Here are some exercise tips to help you feel your best:

- **Go slowly.** It takes time for your body to adjust to anything new. Even if you're an exercise pro, it's a good idea to slow down a little when you first start intermittent fasting to see how your body handles your new routine. If you're new to fasting and exercise, it's even more important to start small—with a few low-intensity workouts each week—and work your way up as you become more fit.
- **Change up your routine.** With fasting, sticking to the same eating schedule is generally best, but the opposite is true of exercise. Doing a mix of different types of workouts and varying your routine through-out the week can help you get rid of body fat and build muscle. Incorporate both low- and high-intensity cardio exercises and strength training.
- **Stay hydrated.** Drinking enough water is always important, but it's even more critical when you're doing fasted exercise. Water helps your muscles grow and repair; when you're dehydrated, it can nega-tively affect your exercise performance. If you're working out first thing in the morning, drink a glass of water before bed, right when you wake up, during your workout, and immediately following.
- **Bump up your electrolytes.** Part of the reason people get dizzy or fatigued from exercise is a loss of electrolytes from sweating. You can replenish those electrolytes naturally with coconut water or natural

sports drinks, like Kill Cliff. These drinks will break your fast, though, so make sure you time them with your eating window.

- **Listen to your body.** Just like there's no one-size-fits-all intermittent fasting schedule, there's no perfect exercise plan that works for everyone. When you exercise, you should feel strong and energized, not burned out and totally depleted. If you feel exhausted after a workout, that's a good sign you're going too hard or not properly fueling your body. Scale back and lower the intensity.
- **Schedule rest days.** Rest days are just as important to physical fitness as active days. Make sure you're scheduling at least one rest day a week to give your body time to repair and recover.

Change Your Protein with Your Exercise Routine

If you're really active or you're in the gym a lot, you may need more protein. It's even possible for your protein needs to change from day to day, based on your activity level. On days when you're working out harder, you'll have higher protein needs than on days when you don't exercise or you do lower-intensity exercises like yoga.

Here are some general protein guidelines:

- **On days when you're not very physically active:** Aim for 0.27–0.45 grams of protein per pound of body weight.
- **On days when you do moderate activity (meaning you exercise on a regular basis but you don't do any high-intensity exercises):** Aim for 0.36–0.45 grams of protein per pound of body weight.
- **On days when you do high-intensity activities (e.g., sprints or bodybuilding):** Aim for 0.45–0.73 grams of protein per pound of body weight. You can start out at 0.45 g/lb and then slowly work your way up and see how you feel.

It's also a good idea to adjust the timing of your protein. Try to spread out your protein intake evenly among your two or three daily meals. This helps ensure that your body can break down and absorb all of the amino acids it needs, since your body can process only about 25–35 grams of protein at a time.

Sleep versus Exercise

Adequate sleep restores your body, repairs your muscles, gives you energy, and helps balance your hormones. And, of course, when you're well rested, it's easier to power through a workout. On the other hand, exercise can boost your energy, improve your mood, contribute to better sleep, and enhance your metabolism.

Sleep and exercise are two of the major foundations of feeling your best, so what do you do when you only have time for one? Most experts agree that you should prioritize sleep. A half hour of exercise is more beneficial healthwise than an extra half hour of sleep, but that's only true if you're getting the base amount of sleep you need—around seven to eight hours. When you're sleep deprived, your body releases inflammatory markers, like C-reactive protein, and bumps up the production of the stress hormones cortisol and adrenaline. If you drag yourself out of bed before your body has had enough rest, you're already off to a bad start hormone-wise.

When you start the day with elevated stress hormones, exercise can turn into a bad stressor, as can fasting, and it can lead to burnout fast. Since this is exactly the thing you're trying to avoid, you need to lay a good foundation for each day with a good night of sleep.

If you're noticing that you're low on energy or you're ending your workouts feeling depleted instead of recharged, you may need more sleep. Of course, the ultimate goal is to go to bed a little bit earlier and wake up a little bit earlier so that you have time for both, but on days when that just isn't possible, don't drag yourself out of bed in the name of exercise.

Taking Targeted Supplements

Sometimes, no matter how good your diet is, you'll still need to take supplements. This can be because you have increased needs for certain nutrients or you live in an area where you don't get enough sunlight.

Exactly which supplements you may need will depend on your specific health and medical history, but some basic supplements that seem to work well for many women include:

- A multivitamin
- Probiotics
- Vitamin D/magnesium

When supplementing with vitamin D, you should also take magnesium, which helps your body convert and absorb vitamin D. Maintaining a proper balance between the two is important for avoiding a deficiency in either, which can have multiple negative health effects.

Some other supplements that are often helpful to feel your best are:

- Protein powder
- Fish oil
- B-complex vitamins
- Adaptogens like ashwagandha, astragalus, cordyceps, rhodiola rosea, and turmeric
- Iron (if you have heavy periods)

It's possible that you have specific deficiencies that could easily be corrected with some targeted supplements. If you suspect that you're deficient in certain nutrients, make an appointment with a functional medicine doctor or a nutritionist who can recommend a specific supplement regimen for you.

Listen to Your Body

Ultimately, the most important thing you can do to make sure you feel good is listen to your body. While there are many theories and science-backed suggestions for improving your health and your mood, you have to do what works for you—and make sure your routine is something that you can stick to long term.

There's an old saying: "One [person]'s meat is another [person]'s poison." Basically, this means that what's good for someone else may not be good for you. This is especially apparent in the case of individual food sensitivities. For example, almonds are technically healthy, but if you have food sensitivity to them, they can act like a poison in your body. This is a prime example of why it's important to listen to what your body is telling you, rather than getting caught up in rigid rules or dietary dogma.

Pay attention to how you feel when you do or eat certain things. If you feel great, continue the course. If you don't feel good, make the necessary changes or adjustments until you do feel good. This does take some time and a lot of self-reflection, but it's entirely worth it. Once you've perfected your program, you're going to be amazed at how great you feel.

Don't Beat Yourself Up

Like anything in life, there can be ups and downs with intermittent fasting. You may feel great one day and then frustrated or tired another, especially in the beginning as your body gets used to it. One of the best things you can do for yourself is understand and accept this.

Avoid getting caught up in perfection and don't expect everything to go smoothly right away. You're going to have bad days; you're going to slip up here and there, and that's okay. If you go into this knowing that you're going to try your best, but that there may be times when it just won't go well, you'll be less likely to beat yourself up when things aren't going according to plan. And being nicer to yourself is a great way to make sure you feel good.

Your Questions Answered

At this point, you have a better understanding about how intermittent fasting works, why women can be more sensitive to it, and how to do it right so that you can reap all of the positive benefits without any of the negatives. But you might still have some lingering questions. Maybe you are wondering whether you should fast during your period. Or you are concerned about possible side effects of fasting.

In this chapter, you'll find answers to some of the most common questions and concerns women have about intermittent fasting. You'll explore the basics of drinking alcohol when fasting, uncover potential reasons for why you may not be losing weight, and more. Keep in mind that these are general answers and do not take the place of medical advice. If you have a specific question or concern about your situation and whether or not fasting will work for you, make sure you discuss it with your doctor before you do anything else.

Will Supplements Break My Fast?

There are many different kinds of supplements out there, so the answer to this question is not a simple yes or no. As a general rule, if a supplement contains macronutrients (carbohydrates, protein, or fat) and/or calories, it can potentially break your fast. Certain ingredients in supplements, like pectin, sugar, fruit juice, and maltodextrin, can also break your fast. If your supplement contains sugar, it's a good idea to swap it out anyway.

Some supplements that can break your fast include:

- Protein powder
- Gummy vitamins or any gummy supplements
- Sweetened liquid supplements
- Branched-chain amino acids
- Collagen

On the other hand, these supplements are usually safe to take during your fast:

- Multivitamins
- Individual micronutrients (vitamin A, vitamin C, calcium, magnesium, etc.)
- Prebiotics and probiotics
- Fish oil
- Creatine

If you're taking supplements, make sure you're following the manufacturer's (or your doctor's) recommendations. Some supplements should be taken first thing in the morning on an empty stomach, while others are absorbed better or better tolerated if you take them with a meal.

Can I Drink Coffee in the Morning?

Here's the good news: You can drink coffee during your fasting window. Here's the (potentially) bad news: You'll have to lose the extra cream and sugar. That means if you're used to drinking a latté or loading your coffee with French vanilla creamer, you'll have to figure out a new way to enjoy coffee if you want to drink it in the early morning hours.

As a general rule, anything that's less than 50 calories won't break your fast, so even if you put a small splash of cream or milk in your coffee, you'll most likely still remain in a fasted state. However, if at all possible, it's best to drink your coffee black. That way, you don't have to worry about the negligible calories that are in coffee without the add-ins.

Black tea, green tea, and herbal tea are also allowed during your fasting window, but the same rule applies: Drink them as is without adding cream and/or sugar. Black tea and green tea are especially good choices because the EGCG (epigallocatechin gallate) in them acts as a caloric restriction mimetic, which means it can help trigger autophagy and boost the effects of your fast.

Be careful not to overdo it, though. While sipping coffee or tea can help control your appetite, too much caffeine, especially on an empty stomach, can leave you feeling jittery and anxious. Caffeine also puts stress on your adrenal glands, so if you're trying to manage your stress and while your body is adjusting to fasting, it's best to limit your intake to one or two cups a day.

Are Diet Sodas Okay to Drink While Fasting?

Because they don't have any carbs or calories, diet sodas can seem like the perfect solution for having a sweet treat while you're fasting. But you know what they say: If it seems too good to be true, it probably is. And that's definitely the case here.

Artificial sweeteners may not have calories, but they disrupt your glucose and insulin levels, increase sugar cravings, and contribute to weight gain by making you feel hungry, increasing sweet cravings, and prompting you to eat more.

It's not only a good idea to avoid artificially sweetened diet sodas while fasting—it's a good idea to avoid them altogether. Keep in mind this only applies to artificial sweeteners, which include:

- Aspartame
- Acesulfame-K
- Sucralose
- Saccharin
- Neotame

Sugar alcohols, like erythritol, and stevia are another story. There are some diet sodas that are sweetened only with stevia and/or erythritol (Virgil's and Zevia are two popular brands). These types of diet sodas, or zero sugar sodas, are okay to drink while fasting since they have no effect on your blood sugar and don't work against autophagy.

That being said, you'll get the most benefit from intermittent fasting if you drink only water, coffee, or tea during your fasting windows. Diet soda, whether sweetened naturally or not, should be only an occasional treat. Even if it doesn't disrupt your blood sugar, it keeps your sugar cravings going strong, and that's not ideal.

Will Intermittent Fasting Make Me Lose Muscle?

One of the biggest concerns surrounding intermittent fasting is that you'll lose lean muscle mass. Many people believe that if you miss a meal, your body will immediately start burning off the protein in your muscles as an energy source, but thanks to human evolution, that's not what happens.

You cannot survive without energy, so even if you don't eat, your body figures out a way to find this energy. Its preferred source is glucose, which comes from either carbohydrates or the glycogen that's stored in your liver or muscles. Its second favorite source is your own body fat, which is essentially excess energy that's been stored for later.

As long as you're eating enough calories, your body knows not to use muscle as its primary energy source and will only use it as a last resort when glucose is depleted and body fat is too low to sustain life. This happens at around 4 percent body fat, which is extremely low. For comparison, female athletes typically have 14–20 percent body fat. So unless you dip below 4 percent body fat, your body will do what it can to preserve lean muscle mass.

It's true that extreme calorie restriction can cause you to lose muscle mass while simultaneously decreasing your metabolism. But remember: Intermittent fasting isn't the same thing as extreme calorie restriction. Studies show that fasting can actually help increase lean muscle mass and help you build muscle instead of breaking it down. That's because when you fast, your body produces more human growth hormone and testosterone and helps improve your insulin sensitivity. This combination of effects helps you build muscle and recover more quickly after exercise.

Isn't Breakfast the Most Important Meal of the Day?

One of the most pervasive nutrition myths is that breakfast is the most important meal of the day. No matter what dietary principles people believe in, many of them still think this is true. But it's not.

One study published in the *British Medical Journal* found that people who ate breakfast consumed more overall calories—260 more per day, to be exact—and weighed more than those who skipped breakfast. The study also found that there were no major differences in metabolic rate between breakfast-eaters and breakfast-skippers. So if you're worried about a negative blow to your metabolism if you skip breakfast, don't be. Another study published in *Nutrients* found that there were no significant differences in weight, metabolism, and nutrient intake in people who eat breakfast versus people who skip it.

But what about all the earlier studies that said eating breakfast helps you lose and maintain weight? Researchers say most of them were observational and the results may have been due to the participants' overall food and lifestyle choices, rather than breakfast itself.

Is Fasting Safe for Women with Thyroid Issues?

There's a common concern that women with thyroid issues shouldn't fast, but it's not fasting itself that's a potential problem. It's calories. When you restrict calories, T4, the inactive thyroid hormone, increases and competes with T3, the active thyroid hormone. This can cause a decrease of up to 50 percent in active T3, which can worsen an existing hypothyroid disease.

But there's evidence that fasting can actually help decrease reliance on thyroid medication and improve fasting insulin and insulin resistance, even if you have hypothyroid issues. If you have a thyroid issue, talk to your doctor before you start, and then do the following:

- **Start slowly.** Begin with shorter fasting protocols like 12/12 and then work your way up to 14/8 if you feel good.
- **Pay extra attention to what you're eating.** Cut out sugar, which can feed the bad bacteria in your gut, and gluten and dairy, which can trigger inflammation and make existing thyroid conditions worse.
- **Don't restrict your calories by more than 20 percent.** For example, if you need 2,000 calories to maintain your weight, don't eat fewer than 1,600 per day.
- **Don't overexercise.** If you're working out too hard, it can have a negative effect on your thyroid, especially when you're fasting too. Keep exercises light, at least in the beginning.
- **Take supplements if you need to.** Selenium, iodine, zinc, and omega-3s are critical for anyone who has thyroid issues.
- **Avoid NSAIDs as much as possible.** NSAIDs, like aspirin and ibuprofen, can lower thyroid hormone concentrations by blocking T4 and T3 from binding with carrier proteins. If you have to take NSAIDs, take them with a meal.

Should I Fast During My Period?

It's perfectly fine to fast during your period; it's the week *before* that you need to be careful about. The week before you start menstruating is when your body is most vulnerable and susceptible to stressors.

During this time, your estrogen levels drop dramatically and you become more sensitive to cortisol, the stress hormone. That's why many women experience symptoms like irritability, low energy, and sugar cravings the week before menstruation starts. Because your body's stress threshold—or ability to respond to and handle stress—lowers during this time, it's possible that fasting can switch from a good stressor to a bad stressor.

This doesn't mean that you have to stop fasting every month, especially if you're feeling good and your stress levels are managed well. It just means you may have to take it a little easier. For example, if you're doing nightly sixteen-hour fasts, scale it back to twelve hours a night. If you're doing alternate-day fasting, you might want to switch to 5:2 (fasting only two days a week instead of every other) just for that week.

What If My Period Stops?

If you stop getting your period and you're not approaching menopause (or going through early menopause), it can be a huge warning sign that there may be something going wrong with your hormones. It can also be an indicator that fasting is acting as a bad stressor, instead of a good one, and that's not what you want.

If this happens, first address your approach to fasting. Are you staying around fourteen to sixteen hours maximum, or have you been doing longer fasts? Are you eating healthy, nutrient-dense meals that provide enough calories, vitamins, and minerals during your eating windows? If your answer to any of these questions is no, change your routine. Scale back on your fasting intensity by reducing the number of hours in your fasting window or, if you're doing daily time-restricted fasting, try fasting every other day instead of every day. When you do eat, focus on eating clean, whole foods and avoid processed foods as much as you can.

If you answered yes to these questions, it's likely that you're dealing with stress overload elsewhere. Stop your fasting plan for now and go back to square one. Work on reducing your stress levels and your overall stress load before trying fasting again.

Keep in mind that changes in your period—like delayed cycles or changes in amount of bleeding—are normal as your body adjusts to intermittent fasting. However, this should all balance out after a couple months. In fact, many women report happier, healthier periods, with fewer cramps and less irritability, after fasting for a while.

Can Fasting Trigger an Eating Disorder?

Many women have expressed concerns about the possibility of fasting triggering an eating disorder or binge-eating behavior. There is evidence that long periods of extreme calorie deprivation can increase the risk of food binges down the line. But remember two things:

1. Intermittent fasting isn't synonymous with calorie restriction. With intermittent fasting, it's recommended that you make sure to get all of the calories you need.
2. While long periods of calorie deprivation may be associated with binge-eating behaviors, the same effect wasn't seen with shorter periods of calorie restriction.

For healthy women without a history of eating disorders, there's no evidence that a properly designed, nutrient-rich intermittent fasting plan will trigger an eating disorder or make binge eating more likely.

The desire to binge is often a result of dramatic dips and surges in blood sugar that occur after a carbohydrate-rich meal. After intermittent fasting for a while, your blood sugar levels tend to stabilize and you have less of a desire to overeat.

If you have a history of disordered eating or you're susceptible to obsessive and/or compulsive behavior around food, it's a good idea to stay away from any form of dietary restriction, including intermittent fasting. If you're concerned about yourself or you're noticing eating patterns or behaviors that you don't like, seek the advice of a health professional.

Why Do I Feel Nauseated in the Morning If I Don't Eat?

Feeling nauseated in the morning is a good sign that your circadian rhythms are off. If you didn't go to bed early enough or you tossed and turned all night, it can mess with your hormones and leave you feeling pretty sick. It's also possible that something you're eating just isn't agreeing with you. This is even more likely if you've made some significant changes to your diet along with adding intermittent fasting.

If you've been intermittent fasting for several weeks and you're still waking up feeling sick in the morning:

- **Check your sleeping habits.** Are you going to bed early enough and getting enough uninterrupted sleep? If not, take a look at your sleeping environment and make the proper changes necessary to get yourself sleeping better. Are you going to bed and waking up at the same time every day?
- **Take stock of what you're eating.** Are there any foods causing digestive upset, bloating, or heartburn? Anything that you're not properly digesting can make you feel nauseated. Pay attention to any foods that seem to repeatedly bother you and then eliminate them for a few weeks to see if that helps.
- **Revisit your stress levels.** Stress and anxiety can make you feel nauseated, even if you don't actually register that you're stressed or anxious. Make sure you're maintaining a self-care routine, outside of fasting, and managing your stress.

Is It Best to Combine Fasting with Keto?

Intermittent fasting and the ketogenic diet go together like peanut butter and jelly—or like eggs and bacon, if you're watching your carbs.

A ketogenic diet is one of three ways (the others are intermittent fasting and exercise) that you can stimulate autophagy. While intermittent fasting requires you to actually go without food, the ketogenic diet essentially tricks the body into thinking it's going without food so that you can experience the same positive metabolic changes. By significantly limiting carbohydrates, you force your body to turn to fat as an energy source. This keeps insulin levels low and glucagon levels high—the perfect combination for stimulating autophagy.

When you combine intermittent fasting and a ketogenic diet, it's like a double whammy for cellular cleansing and fat burn. You're basically turning the heat on full blast, instead of keeping it somewhere on medium.

You can certainly reap all of the benefits of intermittent fasting and autophagy without following a ketogenic diet, though, so it's not a requirement for success. The diet flexibility is actually one of the main reasons many women are drawn to intermittent fasting. It gives more freedom than other eating styles, which makes it easier to stick to long term.

Can I Fast If I Have Hormonal Problems, Like PCOS?

Because one of the concerns about fasting is disruptions in hormones, you might think that if you already have hormonal issues, like polycystic ovary syndrome (PCOS), you're not a good candidate for intermittent fasting. But that's not necessarily true.

Androgen hormones, which include testosterone and androstenedione, are typically thought of as male hormones, but women naturally produce them too, just in smaller amounts. With PCOS, the production of androgen hormones goes up, leading to a hormonal imbalance called hyperandrogenism.

This increased level of androgen hormones causes difficulty getting pregnant, infertility, and/or negative metabolic changes, like insulin resistance, high insulin levels, high cholesterol and triglycerides, and weight gain. There's no single answer as to why some women develop PCOS, but insulin resistance and high insulin levels play a significant role in the hormonal imbalance and the symptoms that come with it.

While mainstream nutrition advice for PCOS is to eat several small meals throughout the day to keep your blood sugar and insulin levels regulated, intermittent fasting actually improves insulin levels—and insulin resistance—better than constantly eating. Studies show that intermittent fasting can reduce insulin growth factor 1, glucose, and insulin levels, which can improve function of the ovaries, decrease androgen hormones, and lessen infertility problems in women with PCOS. And that applies to all forms of intermittent fasting, including alternate-day, time-restricted, 5:2, and spontaneous.

Will Fasting Help with Endometriosis?

As of 2020, there aren't any studies that have directly investigated the effects of fasting on endometriosis, so there's no definitive answer as to whether fasting can help. However, if you look at the underlying causes of endometriosis and fasting's effect on hormones in general, it would be a logical assumption that fasting could at least play a part in helping improve the condition.

While there's no one clear cause of endometriosis, one common characteristic is high estrogen levels or estrogen dominance. This has led medical experts to call it an "estrogen-dependent" disease.

When done right, intermittent fasting has been shown to balance hormones, like estrogen and progesterone. Intermittent fasting also helps improve insulin sensitivity, potentially reversing insulin resistance, which is connected to estrogen dominance and weight gain. And it just so happens that weight gain and obesity are major risk factors for endometriosis.

Managing your stress levels is also extremely important because your body uses up progesterone when producing the stress hormone cortisol. And when progesterone levels are low, you're living in a state of estrogen dominance.

If you have a chronic medical condition, it's always important to discuss any major lifestyle changes with your doctor before starting.

Will Intermittent Fasting Slow My Metabolism?

Unlike low-calorie diets, fasting will not slow down your metabolism. In fact, there are several studies that show that intermittent fasting can actually increase your basal metabolic rate, helping you burn more calories at rest and making it easier for you to maintain weight loss or a healthy weight.

In other words, when you lose weight with intermittent fasting, that weight is more likely to stay off than if you were to lose the same amount of weight by following a low-calorie diet. One study that followed up with *The Biggest Loser* contestants found that their metabolisms were still negatively affected six years later! The problem was that the contestants had followed extremely low-calorie diets, and it's overall calorie restriction, not time-restricted feeding, or fasting, that's more likely to have long-term effects on metabolism. (Confusion around the difference between calorie restriction and fasting is a common theme in many misconceptions about fasting.)

Calorie restriction also drains your energy, which makes it harder to exercise. Studies show that people on low-calorie diets also tend to do less physical activity, which is an important part of maintaining your weight loss. On the flip side, intermittent fasting commonly increases your energy, which makes it more likely that you'll exercise and move around, even if it's just doing chores around the house instead of sitting on the couch binging *Netflix*.

Is There a Best Time of Day to Fast?

When it comes to scheduling your intermittent fast, there's no magic golden hour that will guarantee the best results. However, fasting in the early evening and overnight, then eating earlier in the day, seems to have the most noticeable benefits. As the day goes on, you tend to become more insulin resistant and you don't clear glucose from the blood as efficiently as in the earlier hours.

Studies show that people who eat earlier in the afternoon and evening tend to have a healthier blood lipid profile, and better blood sugar control, and find it easier to maintain a healthy weight than those who eat late at night. On the flip side, people who eat their last meal late at night have blood sugar problems and more difficulty maintaining a healthy weight.

In one study published in *The Journal of Clinical Endocrinology & Metabolism*, researchers had volunteers eat dinner at either 6 p.m. or 10 p.m. and then go to bed at 11 p.m. They found that when participants ate dinner at 10 p.m., their blood sugar levels were higher and they burned less fat, even when the meals were exactly the same.

Research also shows that people who eat late at night tend to make less healthy food choices than those who eat earlier. That bag of chips or those French fries just seem to call out a little louder once it gets dark.

While having dinner at 10 p.m. and then eating your first meal at noon the next day is technically time-restricted fasting, it's probably not the best schedule. Aim to have your last meal between 6 p.m. and 8 p.m. to really reap the full benefits.

Do I Still Have to Count Calories?

You don't have to count calories. That being said, intermittent fasting isn't an excuse to eat all the bad, calorie-dense foods you want during your eating window. Just like you can't exercise your way out of a bad diet, you can't fast your way out of a bad diet either.

While you don't have to log your meals and pay strict attention to your calorie counts, it's still important to make healthy food choices most of the time. Focusing on nutrient-dense foods that come from the earth, avoiding processed foods and sugar, and drinking mostly water will naturally help you stay where you need to be calorie-wise.

In the early stages, it is helpful to log a few days of your diet, using an app like MyFitnessPal or Carb Manager, to get an idea of where you stand and what a proper portion size looks like, but once you have the general idea, you don't have to keep doing it if you don't want to.

How Long Does It Take to Start Seeing Results?

Because every woman is different, this question will have a different answer for everyone. The general consensus is to give intermittent fasting ten to twelve weeks before you make a judgment call on whether or not it's working for you. But that's ten to twelve weeks of consistency. That means really committing to the process and following your intermittent fasting protocol exactly as you scheduled it.

That being said, many women experience results a lot sooner than that. You may start feeling less bloated and weighed down within a couple of days. As the week goes on, you may notice you have more energy and any brain fog and/or sluggishness is starting to lift. And after a couple weeks, you may notice improvements in your skin and feel aches and pains starting to dissipate.

Even if you have a long-term goal, like weight loss, try to focus on these small, gradual improvements in your health as you work toward your larger goal. Celebrating all of the improvements along the way will help make it easier to stick to your plan.

Are There Any Side Effects from Intermittent Fasting?

When you first add intermittent fasting to your lifestyle, it's possible that you'll experience some side effects. These are usually due to blood sugar fluctuations and the most common include:

- Increased hunger
- Cravings, especially for sugar and high-carbohydrate foods
- Irritability
- Light-headedness
- Decreased energy and/or sleepiness
- Weakness
- Headaches

The severity of symptoms can vary based on different factors, like your previous eating habits and how well your body handles insulin, but they shouldn't be severe enough to interfere with your day.

Once your body adapts, typically in about a week or so, these side effects should not only go away, but you should actually start to feel the opposite. For example, fatigue will likely turn into sustained energy, difficulty sleeping will likely turn into nights of restorative uninterrupted sleep, and increased hunger will likely turn into fully feeling satisfied, even if it's been fourteen hours since your last meal.

Keep in mind that while some side effects are normal, you shouldn't be feeling absolutely terrible all the time. If you are, that's a sign that you're going too hard too fast or that you didn't adequately get your stress levels under control before throwing fasting into the mix.

Can I Fast If I Work the Night Shift?

If you're a night shift worker, you probably don't need to be told that that kind of schedule can be really tough on your body. While intermittent fasting may not be able to negate all of the possible negative effects, you can still make it work and reap some of the benefits.

If possible, work your shift into your fasting window so you don't have to eat overnight. Your schedule might look like this:

- **Fasting window:** 11 p.m. to 3 p.m. the next day (work from 11 p.m. to 7 a.m., sleep from when you get home to 3 p.m.)
- **Eating window:** 3 p.m. to 11 p.m.

If you're working longer night-shift hours, this may not work for you. Instead, you can try eating during the morning hours of your shift, instead of in the late-night hours.

Since working the night shift can disrupt your circadian rhythm, even when fasting, it's helpful to eat mostly low-carb, high-fat foods when you do eat. You don't have to follow a ketogenic diet—just a basic low-carb diet would be helpful.

Can I Drink Alcohol While Fasting?

All alcohol has calories, so it will break your fast if you drink it during your fasting window. Drinking on an empty stomach isn't a good idea anyway, since the alcohol can move into your blood more quickly, making you feel intoxicated faster.

If you want to know if you can drink alcohol during your eating window, however, the answer is yes. Eat a meal first and then wait about an hour or so before you begin drinking.

The best alcohol choices are:

- Red or white wine
- Spirits, like vodka, tequila, rum, or whiskey
- Light beer

These alcoholic beverages are lower in carbohydrates and won't spike your blood sugar levels as much as other choices. Just be careful and don't overdo it, especially if you're combining fasting with a ketogenic or low-carb diet. Your alcohol tolerance can go way down when you're not eating many carbs or when you have an empty stomach.

Keep in mind that even though it's okay to drink alcohol during your feeding window, it can still interfere with your metabolism and make it harder to lose weight. If weight loss is one of your major goals, limit your intake as much as possible.

Will Fasting Make My Blood Sugar Too Low?

When you first start intermittent fasting, you may notice symptoms of low blood sugar, like headache, irritability, and hunger. These symptoms can be especially pronounced if you're used to eating a lot of carbohydrates and you've switched to a low-carb diet plan or you have problems with insulin resistance or blood sugar regulation.

While these symptoms can be annoying, in most healthy people, blood sugar won't get low enough to warrant an actual problem. Your body has built-in physiological mechanisms that keep your blood sugar levels within a certain range so you don't pass out or experience any other serious health problems.

As time goes on and you become more sensitive to insulin and get off the blood sugar roller coaster you've been on, your body adjusts and your blood sugar will be maintained even more tightly. When this happens, you likely won't experience any symptoms, even hunger, during your fasting time.

This doesn't apply if you have diabetes, though. If you're a type 1 diabetic, you should absolutely not do any form of fasting without permission, and close monitoring, from your doctor. There are some studies that show type 1 diabetics were able to lower their insulin doses after sticking with a fasting plan for a period of time, but if you don't do it right or you don't ease into it properly and combine fasting with the right types of foods, it can lead to dangerously low blood sugar levels.

Do I Have to Eat If I'm Not Hungry?

If you're used to hearing that you need to eat several small meals through-out the day to keep your metabolism stoked, it may be hard to retrain your brain to be okay with going without meals. But if your feeding window has arrived and you don't feel hungry, you don't *have* to eat.

Of course, you don't want to restrict your overall daily calories too much and you don't want to go too long without eating. It's okay to delay your meal an hour or two, but if you're still not feeling hungry sixteen to eighteen hours into your fast, it's probably a good idea to eat something.

You don't have to force a big meal down, though. Sipping on a veg-etable soup or drinking a macronutrient-balanced smoothie can be a good way to break your fast when you don't really have an appetite.

Why Am I Not Losing Weight?

If weight loss is one of your major goals, it can be extremely frustrating when you're not seeing results on the scale. The first thing you need to do is be patient. Weight loss can take time—usually more time than you'd like—but if you stay consistent, it should happen.

If you've been intermittent fasting for a while and you're still not losing weight, some things that can help are:

- **Cleaning up your diet.** While you can see some serious benefits with intermittent fasting alone, it's always a good idea to clean up your diet, especially if you want to lose weight. Cut out processed foods and sugar, eat more vegetables, and switch to high-quality meats.
- **Drinking more water.** Aim for at least half of your body weight in ounces.
- **Making sure you're not consuming any artificial sweeteners.** Check your labels and avoid anything with sucralose, aspartame, acesulfame-K, saccharin, advantame, and neotame.
- **Checking your stress levels.** Is stress creeping up on you again? If so, make sure you're incorporating the appropriate stress reduction techniques and practicing them daily, even when you feel good physically.
- **Scaling back on your intensity.** If you're currently fasting every other day or doing daily fourteen- to sixteen-hour fasts, try scaling back to a couple times a week or twelve-hour fasts to see if your body responds to that better.

Is It Normal to Feel Hungry All the Time?

There's no way to predict exactly how you'll feel when you first start intermittent fasting; every woman is different. If you're used to eating five or six times during the day or late into the night, it's highly likely that you'll feel hungry during your fasting window for the first several weeks. You'll probably have more intense cravings too. Often, this is emotional or mental hunger, rather than true physical hunger.

After the first few weeks, as your body adjusts, your blood sugar and insulin levels begin to stabilize, and that's where all the good stuff happens. Your hunger will likely go away, and you should feel sustained energy throughout the day.

However, if you've been following an intermittent fasting protocol for several weeks and you still feel hungry all the time, you'll probably have to do some troubleshooting:

- Calculate your calorie needs and then track your food for a few days to make sure you're hitting them. If you're way under, increase your portion sizes.
- Make sure you're eating enough healthy fats; they're essential to keeping you feeling full. Add avocados, olives, olive oil, grass-fed butter, ghee, fatty fish, nuts, and seeds to your meals.
- Check your protein intake. You should be eating around 0.8–1.0 gram of protein per kilogram of body weight.
- Drink more water. Sometimes thirst is disguised as hunger.

Can I Take the Weekends Off?

One of the great things about intermittent fasting is the flexibility it offers. Part of that flexibility is adjusting your fasting schedule when you have social events or things that you want to do on the weekend.

If you're really social and outgoing and the thought of having to fast on the weekends is keeping you from diving in, design your fasting plan around that. You can do the 5:2 method and fast on Tuesday and Thursday, or you can do a Tuesday, Thursday, Saturday alternate-day fasting schedule and fast only on one weekend day. You can even do fourteen-hour time-restricted fasts all week and then take the weekends off.

Of course, the more you stick to the plan and make good choices, even on the weekend, the better your results will be. But intermittent fasting is meant to be a lifestyle; to stick with it long term, it can't feel like a prison sentence. You have to be able to fit it in with the other things you enjoy doing.

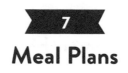

Meal Plans

One of the best things about intermittent fasting is that you can incorporate it into any lifestyle. There are no strict diet or food rules to follow, so you can make it work for you no matter what your dietary preferences are. In this chapter, you'll find ketogenic, low-carb, Paleo, gluten-free, clean eating, vegetarian, and vegan meal plans that utilize common ingredients you can find in most grocery stores. You'll also see easy recipes that can be incorporated into different plans, as well as some suggestions of clean brands that taste great with minimal ingredients. You can follow the meal plans exactly as they're written or mix and match meal ideas to create a food plan that works for you.

Remember: Intermittent fasting isn't meant to be a low-calorie diet, so these meal plans don't have strict quantities or portions. The goal is to make sure you're meeting your specific calorie needs and getting enough nutrients every day, without going overboard.

Intermittent Fasting Recipes

The following are delicious, easy-to-make recipes you can incorporate into your intermittent fasting schedule. Each recipe is labeled to show in which of the different meal plans presented at the end of this chapter they are used.

Chocolate Fat Bomb Smoothie

`KETO`

Serves 1

1 cup unsweetened vanilla almond milk
1 teaspoon MCT oil
1 scoop keto-friendly chocolate protein powder

Combine all ingredients in a blender. Blend and serve immediately.

Two-Ingredient Chaffles

`KETO`

Serves 1

1 large egg
½ cup shredded mozzarella cheese

1. Preheat mini waffle iron.
2. Combine egg and cheese in a medium bowl and whisk until combined.
3. Pour half the mixture onto preheated waffle iron. Cook for 3 minutes or until golden brown. Remove from heat.
4. Repeat with remaining batter.
5. Serve immediately.

Chocolate Chaffles

KETO

Serves 1

1 large egg
½ cup shredded mozzarella cheese
1 tablespoon unsweetened cocoa powder
1 teaspoon powdered erythritol

1. Preheat mini waffle iron.
2. Combine ingredients in a medium bowl and whisk until combined.
3. Pour half the mixture onto preheated waffle iron. Cook for 3 minutes or until golden brown. Remove from heat.
4. Repeat with remaining batter.
5. Serve immediately.

Overnight "Oats"

LOW-CARB

Serves 1

1½ tablespoons chia seeds

1½ tablespoons hemp hearts

1 tablespoon unsweetened shredded coconut

¾ cup unsweetened almond milk

2 tablespoons plain Greek yogurt

1 teaspoon powdered erythritol

1 tablespoon chopped walnuts

1. Combine all ingredients in a glass Mason jar, cover, and shake vigorously until blended.
2. Refrigerate for 4 hours or overnight.
3. Serve chilled.

Chocolate Strawberry Smoothie

PALEO

Serves 1

1 cup unsweetened almond milk

¾ cup frozen sliced strawberries

1 scoop Paleo chocolate protein powder (such as Designs for Health)

½ cup frozen chopped kale

1 tablespoon melted coconut oil

Combine all ingredients in a blender. Blend until smooth and serve immediately.

Paleo Pancakes

PALEO

Serves 1

1 tablespoon butter-flavored coconut oil
¼ cup almond flour
2 tablespoons coconut flour
2 tablespoons tapioca flour
2 teaspoons maple sugar
¼ teaspoon baking soda
⅛ teaspoon fine sea salt
2 large eggs, lightly beaten
2 tablespoons unsweetened vanilla almond milk
1 teaspoon white wine vinegar
1 teaspoon vanilla extract

1. Heat coconut oil in a medium skillet over low heat.
2. Combine almond flour, coconut flour, tapioca flour, sugar, baking soda, and salt in a sifter and sift into a medium bowl. Set aside.
3. Combine remaining ingredients in a separate medium bowl.
4. Pour wet ingredients into dry ingredients and mix until just blended.
5. Spoon about 2 tablespoons of batter onto preheated skillet and cook for 2 minutes on each side. Repeat with remaining batter.
6. Serve with maple syrup or topping of choice.

Chocolate Peanut Butter Smoothie

KETO

Serves 1

1 cup unsweetened chocolate almond milk

1 scoop keto-friendly chocolate protein powder

2 tablespoons no-sugar-added peanut butter

2 teaspoons MCT oil

1 teaspoon powdered erythritol

½ cup ice

> Combine all ingredients in a blender and blend until smooth. Serve immediately.

Chocolate Strawberry Overnight Oats

GLUTEN-FREE

Serves 1

¼ cup gluten-free quick-cooking rolled oats

½ cup unsweetened vanilla almond milk

3 strawberries, stemmed and sliced

1 tablespoon pure maple syrup

1 tablespoon stevia-sweetened chocolate chips (such as Lily's)

1. Combine all ingredients in a glass Mason jar, cover, and shake vigorously until blended.
2. Refrigerate for 4 hours or overnight.
3. Serve chilled.

Chocolate Chia Pudding

GLUTEN-FREE

Serves 1

¼ cup unsweetened cashew milk

¼ cup chilled brewed coffee

2 teaspoons cashew butter

½ teaspoon vanilla extract

1 tablespoon pure maple syrup

2 teaspoons unsweetened cocoa powder

2 tablespoons chia seeds

1. Combine all ingredients, except chia seeds, in a glass Mason jar, cover, and shake vigorously until blended.
2. Add chia seeds, close jar, and shake again.
3. Refrigerate overnight and serve chilled.

Mixed Berry Smoothie

VEGAN

Serves 1

¾ cup unsweetened almond milk

¼ cup unsweetened banana milk

¾ cup frozen mixed berries

1 scoop vegan protein powder

½ cup chopped spinach

1 tablespoon melted coconut oil

    Combine all ingredients in a blender. Blend until smooth and serve immediately.

Pumpkin Walnut Overnight Oats

VEGETARIAN **VEGAN**

Serves 1

¼ cup quick-cooking rolled oats

½ cup unsweetened vanilla almond milk

3 tablespoons pumpkin purée

2 tablespoons chopped walnuts

1 tablespoon pure maple syrup

⅛ teaspoon pumpkin pie spice

1. Combine all ingredients in a glass Mason jar, cover, and shake vigorously until blended.
2. Refrigerate for 4 hours or overnight.
3. Serve chilled.

Banana Chia Pudding

CLEAN EATING

Serves 1

¼ cup full-fat coconut milk

¼ cup banana milk

2 teaspoons almond butter

½ teaspoon vanilla extract

1 tablespoon pure maple syrup

2 tablespoons chia seeds

1. Combine all ingredients, except chia seeds, in a glass Mason jar, cover, and shake vigorously until blended.
2. Add chia seeds, close jar, and shake again.
3. Refrigerate overnight and serve chilled.

Anti-Inflammatory Smoothie

CLEAN EATING **VEGAN**

Serves 1

1 cup unsweetened almond milk
½ medium banana, peeled and frozen
1 scoop vanilla protein powder (such as Tera's Whey)
1 scoop superspice mix (such as California Gold Dust)
1 tablespoon melted coconut oil
2 raw Brazil nuts

Combine all ingredients in a blender. Blend until smooth.

Banana Walnut Overnight Oats

CLEAN EATING

Serves 1

¼ cup quick-cooking rolled oats
½ cup unsweetened vanilla almond milk
3 tablespoons mashed banana
2 tablespoons crushed walnuts
1 tablespoon pure maple syrup
⅛ teaspoon ground cinnamon

1. Combine all ingredients in a glass Mason jar, cover, and shake vigorously until blended.
2. Refrigerate for 4 hours or overnight.
3. Serve chilled.

Tofu Scramble

VEGAN

Serves 1

1 teaspoon olive oil

¼ teaspoon minced garlic

1 tablespoon minced yellow onion

1 (8-ounce) block firm tofu, mashed

1 tablespoon nutritional yeast

⅛ teaspoon garlic powder

⅛ teaspoon turmeric

1 tablespoon unsweetened oat milk

¼ cup finely chopped broccoli

¼ small avocado, peeled, pitted, and sliced

1. Heat olive oil in a medium skillet over medium heat.
2. Add minced garlic and onion and sauté until softened, about 3 minutes.
3. Add tofu and cook for 5 minutes, or until most of the water has evaporated.
4. Stir in nutritional yeast, garlic powder, and turmeric and continue cooking for another 4 minutes.
5. Stir in oat milk and cook for 1 minute.
6. Add broccoli and cook until softened, about 3 more minutes.
7. Remove from heat, top with avocado slices, and serve.

PB&J Overnight Oats

VEGAN

Serves 1

¼ cup quick-cooking rolled oats

½ cup unsweetened oat milk

3 tablespoons no-sugar-added peanut butter

¼ cup mashed fresh or thawed frozen strawberries

1 tablespoon pure maple syrup

1. Combine all ingredients in a glass Mason jar, cover, and shake vigorously until blended.
2. Refrigerate for 4 hours or overnight.
3. Serve chilled.

Chocolate Strawberry Chia Pudding

VEGETARIAN

Serves 1

½ cup unsweetened chocolate oat milk

2 teaspoons almond butter

½ teaspoon vanilla extract

1 tablespoon pure maple syrup

¼ cup mashed fresh or thawed frozen strawberries

2 tablespoons chia seeds

1. Combine all ingredients, except chia seeds, in a glass Mason jar, cover, and shake vigorously until blended.
2. Add chia seeds, close jar, and shake again.
3. Refrigerate overnight and serve chilled.

Cinnamon Apple Quinoa Bowl

VEGETARIAN

Serves 1

¾ cup unsweetened almond milk

⅔ cup diced apples

¼ cup quinoa

¼ teaspoon ground cinnamon

⅛ teaspoon ground nutmeg

⅛ teaspoon fine sea salt

1 teaspoon pure maple syrup

1 tablespoon sliced almonds

1. Combine all ingredients, except almonds, in a small saucepan. Bring to a boil over medium-high heat. Reduce heat to low, cover, and simmer for 10 minutes or until liquid is absorbed.
2. Remove from heat and let sit for 5 minutes.
3. Transfer to a serving bowl and sprinkle sliced almonds on top. Serve immediately.

Meal Plans

KETO MEAL PLAN

DAY 1	
Breakfast	Chocolate Fat Bomb Smoothie (see recipe)
Lunch	3 slices no-sugar-added deli turkey layered with 3 slices American cheese, ¼ cup thinly sliced cucumber, and ¼ teaspoon lemon pepper
Dinner	½ cup cooked taco meat topped with 2 tablespoons shredded Cheddar cheese, 1 teaspoon sour cream, 1 tablespoon chopped black olives, chopped lettuce, chopped fresh cilantro, and ⅛ teaspoon hot sauce
Snack	1 cheese stick
DAY 2	
Breakfast	2 scrambled eggs, 2 no-sugar-added sausage links, and ¼ medium avocado (sliced)
Lunch	1 cup chopped lettuce topped with ½ can wild-caught tuna mixed with 1 tablespoon mayonnaise, 2 tablespoons diced cucumber, 2 tablespoons diced tomato, and 1 tablespoon shredded Cheddar cheese
Dinner	1 cup zucchini noodles topped with ¼ cup homemade Alfredo sauce and 1 tablespoon grated Parmesan cheese
Snack	½ medium avocado (sliced), sprinkled with sea salt, pepper, and ¼ teaspoon hot sauce
DAY 3	
Breakfast	Two-Ingredient Chaffles (see recipe) topped with ½ medium avocado (mashed) and sprinkled with Everything but the Bagel seasoning
Lunch	3 chopped hard-boiled eggs mixed with 1 tablespoon mayonnaise and eaten with ⅓ cup sliced zucchini
Dinner	1 cup chopped lettuce topped with ½ cup cooked chicken breast, 1 tablespoon crumbled feta cheese, ¼ medium avocado (sliced), 1 tablespoon diced red onion, and 2 tablespoons keto-friendly dressing of your choice
Snack	2 medium celery stalks filled with cream cheese

DAY 4	
Breakfast	2 over-easy eggs over ½ cup sautéed spinach and sliced mushrooms, sprinkled with 1 tablespoon Parmesan cheese
Lunch	¼ cup cubed no-sugar-added ham, ¼ cup cubed turkey, ¼ cup cubed Swiss cheese, ¼ cup cubed Cheddar cheese tossed together and topped with 2 tablespoons Italian dressing
Dinner	1 (4-ounce) baked salmon fillet with ½ cup roasted broccoli tossed in 2 teaspoons olive oil
Snack	1 ounce cubed cheese (any variety) with 1 ounce macadamia nuts

DAY 5	
Breakfast	2 scrambled eggs with 2 tablespoons shredded Cheddar cheese and 3 pieces no-sugar-added bacon
Lunch	½ can wild-caught tuna combined with 1 tablespoon mayonnaise and served on romaine lettuce boats topped with ¼ medium avocado (sliced)
Dinner	1 (4-ounce) ribeye steak topped with 2 tablespoons crumbled blue cheese and 6 stalks asparagus
Snack	½ cucumber (sliced) with 2 tablespoons ranch dressing

DAY 6	
Breakfast	2 Chocolate Chaffles (see recipe) topped with 1 tablespoon grass-fed butter and 1 tablespoon ChocZero chocolate syrup
Lunch	½ cup cubed cooked chicken thighs, 2 tablespoons shredded Cheddar cheese, 1 tablespoon chopped black olives, and ¼ medium avocado (sliced) topped with hot sauce
Dinner	1 cup zucchini noodles with 2 tablespoons homemade garlic butter sauce topped with ¾ cup cooked medium shrimp
Snack	1 Epic meat bar

DAY 7	
Breakfast	Chocolate Peanut Butter Smoothie (see recipe)
Lunch	½ cup shredded cooked chicken mixed with 1 tablespoon mayonnaise and served with ¼ medium avocado (sliced) sprinkled with Everything but the Bagel seasoning
Dinner	1 (4-ounce) chicken thigh with ¼ cup cauliflower rice and ½ cup spinach and sliced mushrooms sautéed in 1 tablespoon garlic butter
Snack	2 hard-boiled eggs

LOW-CARB MEAL PLAN

DAY 1	
Breakfast	¼ cup plain Greek yogurt topped with 1 tablespoon sliced almonds, ¼ cup wild blueberries, and ⅛ teaspoon ground cinnamon
Lunch	½ cup cooked chicken breast with ¼ cup chopped cucumber, ¼ cup cherry tomatoes, 1 tablespoon diced red onion, ¼ medium avocado (cubed), chopped fresh cilantro, and 1 tablespoon Italian dressing
Dinner	1 (4-ounce) baked cod fillet with 1 tablespoon butter on top of 1 cup lightly steamed zucchini noodles
Snack	2 tablespoons unsweetened cashew butter with 1 tablespoon Lily's stevia-sweetened chocolate chips
DAY 2	
Breakfast	Overnight "Oats" (see recipe)
Lunch	1 cup baby kale topped with ½ cup mixed berries, ¼ cup crumbled feta cheese, and ½ cup cooked cubed steak
Dinner	1 (4-ounce) grilled chicken breast with ½ cup roasted butternut squash and ½ cup mashed cauliflower
Snack	½ medium zucchini (sliced) with ⅓ cup marinara sauce, 24 mini pepperoni slices, and ¼ cup shredded mozzarella cheese (broiled until cheese is melted)
DAY 3	
Breakfast	3-egg omelet with ½ cup spinach, 1 tablespoon diced yellow onion, and 1 tablespoon crumbled feta cheese
Lunch	2 hard-boiled eggs mashed with ¼ medium avocado, 1 strip crumbled bacon, 1 tablespoon mayonnaise, and salt and pepper to taste, served over lettuce leaves or with ½ medium zucchini (sliced)
Dinner	1 (4-ounce) sirloin steak with ½ cup steamed broccoli and cauliflower tossed in 1 tablespoon olive oil and sprinkled with chunky sea salt
Snack	1 cheese stick with 4 Brazil nuts
DAY 4	
Breakfast	½ cup plain Greek yogurt topped with ¼ cup chopped strawberries, 1 tablespoon drizzled peanut butter, and 1 teaspoon Lily's stevia-sweetened chocolate chips

Lunch	2 cups mixed greens topped with ½ can tuna (drained), ¼ medium avocado (sliced), 3 sliced strawberries, 1 tablespoon sliced almonds, 1 tablespoon crumbled feta cheese, and 1 tablespoon Tessemae's honey poppyseed dressing
Dinner	1 (4-ounce) roasted chicken breast with ½ cup roasted garlic broccoli tossed in 1 tablespoon olive oil and a sprinkle of sea salt
Snack	1 Country Archer Original Beef Stick
DAY 5	
Breakfast	1 Cali'flour Foods flatbread, toasted and topped with ¼ medium avocado (mashed), 1 tablespoon crumbled feta cheese, and ⅛ teaspoon Everything but the Bagel seasoning
Lunch	Leftover chicken and roasted garlic broccoli with ½ cup cauliflower rice
Dinner	1 cup cooked spaghetti squash topped with ½ cup marinara sauce, 1 sliced chicken sausage, and 1 tablespoon grated Parmesan cheese
Snack	⅓ cup feta-stuffed green olives
DAY 6	
Breakfast	2 scrambled eggs with ½ cup pan-fried shredded zucchini and 2 slices no-sugar-added bacon
Lunch	3 romaine lettuce leaves topped with 1 chopped hard-boiled egg, 2 tablespoons shredded Cheddar cheese, ¼ cup chopped tomato, ¼ medium avocado (chopped), and 2 slices bacon (chopped) drizzled with 1 tablespoon ranch dressing
Dinner	1 (4-ounce) broiled salmon fillet with 7 stalks herb-roasted asparagus and ½ cup cauliflower rice
Snack	1 medium pear with 2 ounces Cheddar cheese
DAY 7	
Breakfast	1 cup coconut milk, ¼ cup frozen spinach, ¼ medium avocado, 2 scoops vanilla protein powder, and 1 tablespoon hempseeds blended until smooth
Lunch	4 slices roasted deli turkey, ¼ medium avocado (sliced), ½ cup fresh spinach, and 1 tablespoon crumbled feta cheese on 2 Outer Aisle cauliflower sandwich thins
Dinner	3 iceberg lettuce leaves topped with ½ cup ground taco meat, 1 tablespoon sour cream, 2 tablespoons shredded Mexican-style cheese, ¼ cup salsa, and 2 tablespoons sliced black olives
Snack	½ medium zucchini (sliced) with ¼ cup guacamole

PALEO MEAL PLAN

DAY 1

Breakfast	2 Teton Waters Ranch breakfast sausages and 2 fried eggs served over ¼ cup sautéed spinach and minced yellow onion
Lunch	1 (4-ounce) baked salmon fillet with ½ cup roasted broccoli tossed in 1 tablespoon olive oil
Dinner	1 cup zucchini noodles topped with 1 (4-ounce) baked chicken breast, ⅓ cup marinara sauce, and ¼ cup sliced roasted mushrooms
Snack	½ medium avocado (sliced), sprinkled with sea salt, pepper, and ¼ teaspoon hot sauce

DAY 2

Breakfast	1 medium mashed sweet potato, ⅓ cup chopped chorizo, 2 chopped hard-boiled eggs, and ¼ medium avocado (chopped) mixed together
Lunch	3 chopped hard-boiled eggs mixed with 1 tablespoon Tessemae's mayonnaise and eaten with ½ medium zucchini (sliced) or ½ cup plantain chips
Dinner	1 (4-ounce) baked garlic chicken breast with ½ cup cauliflower rice and ½ cup roasted green beans
Snack	1 medium apple with 2 tablespoons almond butter

DAY 3

Breakfast	Chocolate Strawberry Smoothie (see recipe)
Lunch	½ can wild-caught tuna with 1 tablespoon mayonnaise served on romaine lettuce boats topped with ¼ medium avocado (sliced)
Dinner	1 large baked sweet potato stuffed with ⅓ cup cooked ground beef, ½ cup sautéed kale, and ¼ medium avocado (sliced) drizzled with 1 tablespoon Tessemae's avocado ranch dressing
Snack	1 Country Archer Original Beef Stick

DAY 4

Breakfast	3 eggs scrambled with ⅓ cup sliced mushrooms and minced yellow onion, and served with ¼ cup diced roasted sweet potatoes and 2 slices no-sugar-added bacon
Lunch	1 medium avocado halved and stuffed with ½ cup tuna salad
Dinner	3 iceberg lettuce leaves stuffed with ⅓ cup ground taco meat, ¼ cup salsa, ¼ medium avocado (sliced), and 1 tablespoon sliced black olives and drizzled with 2 tablespoons Tessemae's habanero ranch dressing

Snack	1 Lärabar
DAY 5	
Breakfast	Paleo Pancakes (see recipe) with 2 tablespoons almond butter and 2 tablespoons pure maple syrup
Lunch	2 cups chopped romaine lettuce topped with 1 (4-ounce) cooked chicken breast, ¼ cup black beans, 2 tablespoons diced bell peppers, ¼ cup grape tomatoes, ¼ cup chopped avocado, 1 tablespoon black olives, and 1 tablespoon crushed plantain chips drizzled with 2 tablespoons Tessemae's avocado ranch dressing
Dinner	1 cup zucchini noodles with ¼ cup homemade garlic ghee sauce topped with ¾ cup cooked medium shrimp
Snack	1 Epic meat bar
DAY 6	
Breakfast	1 (4-ounce) cooked steak with 2 over-easy eggs and ⅓ cup sautéed diced zucchini
Lunch	½ cup cauliflower rice with ⅓ cup ground turkey and ½ cup steamed broccoli topped with Wildbrine Spicy Kimchi Sriracha
Dinner	1 Cali'flour plant-based Italian pizza crust with ¼ cup pizza sauce, 2¼ cups mozzarella cheese, and 8 nitrate-free pepperoni slices and a side salad
Snack	¼ cup Brazil nuts
DAY 7	
Breakfast	2 scrambled eggs with ½ medium avocado (sliced), drizzled with 1 teaspoon hot sauce, and 3 pieces no-sugar-added bacon
Lunch	½ cup cubed cooked chicken thighs, ½ cup cauliflower rice, 1 tablespoon chopped black olives, and ¼ medium avocado (sliced) mixed and topped with hot sauce
Dinner	1 Teton Waters Ranch burger served on 1 cup chopped romaine lettuce with 1 tablespoon chopped yellow onion and 1 tablespoon chopped pickles and drizzled with 1 tablespoon Tessemae's ketchup, 2 teaspoons mustard, and 1 tablespoon Tessemae's mayonnaise
Snack	1 medium banana (sliced) topped with 1 tablespoon melted coconut butter and 1 tablespoon unsweetened shredded coconut

GLUTEN-FREE MEAL PLAN

DAY 1	
Breakfast	¼ cup plain Greek yogurt topped with 1 tablespoon crushed walnuts, ½ medium banana (sliced), and ⅛ teaspoon ground cinnamon
Lunch	2 cups chopped romaine lettuce topped with 1 (4-ounce) cooked chicken breast, ¼ cup black beans, ¼ cup chopped bell peppers, ¼ cup grape tomatoes, ¼ medium avocado (chopped), 1 tablespoon sliced black olives, and 1 tablespoon crushed plantain chips; add 2 tablespoons gluten-free dressing of your choice
Dinner	1 Cali'flour pizza crust with ¼ cup pizza sauce, ¼ cup mozzarella cheese, and 8 nitrate-free pepperoni slices and a side salad
Snack	½ medium avocado (sliced) sprinkled with sea salt, black pepper, and ¼ teaspoon hot sauce
DAY 2	
Breakfast	3-egg omelet with ½ cup spinach and minced yellow onion, and 1 tablespoon crumbled feta cheese
Lunch	4 slices roasted deli turkey, ¼ medium avocado (chopped), ½ cup fresh spinach, and 1 tablespoon crumbled feta cheese on 2 pieces Outer Aisle cauliflower sandwich thins
Dinner	1 cup zucchini noodles topped with 1 (4-ounce) baked chicken breast, ¼ cup marinara sauce, and 1 tablespoon grated Parmesan cheese
Snack	2 tablespoons unsweetened cashew butter with 1 tablespoon Lily's stevia-sweetened chocolate chips
DAY 3	
Breakfast	Chocolate Strawberry Overnight Oats (see recipe)
Lunch	1 large gluten-free tortilla with 2 tablespoons refried beans, ¼ cup salsa, ½ medium avocado (sliced), chopped fresh cilantro, and hot sauce
Dinner	1 Teton Waters Ranch burger served on ½ cup chopped romaine lettuce with 1 tablespoon minced yellow onion and 1 tablespoon minced pickles, drizzled with 1 tablespoon Tessemae's ketchup, 2 teaspoons mustard, and 1 tablespoon Tessemae's mayonnaise
Snack	¾ cup Siete grain-free lime tortilla chips with ¼ cup guacamole
DAY 4	
Breakfast	3 eggs scrambled with ½ cup sliced mushrooms and minced yellow onion and served with ½ cup diced roasted sweet potatoes and 2 slices no-sugar-added bacon

Lunch	½ cup cubed cooked chicken thighs, 2 tablespoons shredded Cheddar cheese, 1 tablespoon chopped black olives, and ¼ medium avocado (sliced) mixed and topped with hot sauce
Dinner	1 cup lightly cooked zucchini noodles with ¼ cup homemade garlic butter sauce topped with ¾ cup cooked medium shrimp
Snack	½ medium zucchini (sliced) with 2 tablespoons Tessemae's avocado ranch dressing
DAY 5	
Breakfast	½ cup plain Greek yogurt topped with 6 chopped strawberries, 1 tablespoon drizzled peanut butter, and 1 teaspoon Lily's stevia-sweetened chocolate chips
Lunch	4 ounces baked salmon with ½ cup roasted broccoli tossed in 1 tablespoon olive oil
Dinner	½ cup cooked taco meat topped with 1 tablespoon shredded Cheddar cheese, 1 tablespoon sour cream, 1 tablespoon sliced black olives, ½ cup chopped lettuce, chopped fresh cilantro, and ⅛ teaspoon hot sauce
Snack	2 cups air-popped popcorn sprinkled with 2 teaspoons nutritional yeast
DAY 6	
Breakfast	½ cup cooked gluten-free oatmeal topped with ½ medium banana (sliced), ¼ cup crushed walnuts, 1 tablespoon maple syrup, and ⅛ teaspoon ground cinnamon
Lunch	3 chopped hard-boiled eggs mixed with 1 tablespoon mayonnaise and eaten with ½ medium zucchini (sliced) or ⅓ cup plantain chips
Dinner	¼ cup cooked quinoa mixed with ¼ cup ground turkey, ¼ cup chopped tomato, ¼ cup sliced roasted mushrooms, and ¼ cup roasted asparagus
Snack	½ cup fresh raspberries with 1 ounce organic dark chocolate
DAY 7	
Breakfast	Chocolate Chia Pudding (see recipe)
Lunch	1 cup chopped lettuce topped with ½ can wild-caught tuna mixed with 1 tablespoon mayonnaise, ¼ cup diced cucumber, ¼ cup diced tomato, and 1 tablespoon shredded Cheddar cheese
Dinner	2 Outer Aisle cauliflower sandwich thins with ¼ cup pizza sauce, ¼ cup fresh mozzarella cheese chunks, fresh basil, and 4 tomato slices
Snack	12 gluten-free crackers with 2 ounces sharp Cheddar cheese

CLEAN EATING MEAL PLAN

DAY 1	
Breakfast	¼ cup plain Greek yogurt topped with 6 sliced strawberries, ½ small banana (sliced), and ⅛ teaspoon ground cinnamon
Lunch	1 large gluten-free tortilla with 2 tablespoons refried beans, ¼ cup salsa, ¼ medium avocado (sliced), chopped fresh cilantro, and hot sauce
Dinner	1 (4-ounce) baked salmon fillet with ½ cup roasted broccoli tossed in 1 tablespoon olive oil
Snack	1 small banana (sliced) with 2 tablespoons peanut butter
DAY 2	
Breakfast	Banana Chia Pudding (see recipe)
Lunch	½ cup cubed cooked chicken thighs, 2 tablespoons shredded Cheddar cheese, 1 tablespoon chopped black olives, and ¼ medium avocado (sliced) mixed and topped with hot sauce
Dinner	1 Teton Waters Ranch burger served on 1 cup chopped romaine lettuce with 1 tablespoon minced yellow onion and 1 tablespoon chopped pickles and drizzled with 1 tablespoon Tessemae's ketchup, 2 teaspoons mustard, and 1 tablespoon Tessemae's mayonnaise
Snack	12 gluten-free crackers with 2 ounces sharp Cheddar cheese
DAY 3	
Breakfast	3 eggs scrambled with ½ cup sliced mushrooms and minced yellow onion and served with ½ cup diced roasted sweet potatoes and 2 slices no-sugar-added bacon
Lunch	2 slices gluten-free toast spread with 2 tablespoons hummus and topped with ½ small cucumber (sliced), ¼ cup diced tomato, ¼ cup chopped spinach, and ⅛ teaspoon lemon pepper
Dinner	½ cup cooked taco meat topped with 1 tablespoon shredded Cheddar cheese, 1 tablespoon sour cream, 1 tablespoon sliced black olives, ¼ cup chopped lettuce, fresh cilantro, and ⅛ teaspoon hot sauce
Snack	1 RX Bar
DAY 4	
Breakfast	½ cup plain Greek yogurt topped with ½ small banana (chopped), 1 tablespoon drizzled peanut butter, and 1 teaspoon Lily's stevia-sweetened chocolate chips

Lunch	1 cup chopped lettuce topped with ½ can wild-caught tuna mixed with 1 tablespoon mayonnaise, ¼ cup diced cucumber, ¼ cup diced tomato, and 1 tablespoon shredded Cheddar cheese
Dinner	1 cup zucchini noodles with ¼ cup homemade garlic butter sauce, topped with ¾ cup cooked medium shrimp
Snack	¼ cup Brazil nuts
DAY 5	
Breakfast	Anti-Inflammatory Smoothie (see recipe)
Lunch	¼ cup cubed no-sugar-added ham, ¼ cup cubed turkey, ¼ cup cubed Swiss cheese, and ¼ cup cubed Cheddar cheese tossed and topped with 2 tablespoons Italian dressing
Dinner	2 Outer Aisle cauliflower sandwich thins topped with ¼ cup pizza sauce, ¼ cup fresh mozzarella cheese chunks, fresh basil, and 4 tomato slices
Snack	2 cups air-popped popcorn sprinkled with 2 teaspoons nutritional yeast
DAY 6	
Breakfast	3-egg omelet with ⅓ cup spinach, 1 tablespoon minced yellow onion, and 2 tablespoons crumbled feta cheese
Lunch	4 slices roasted deli turkey, ¼ medium avocado (sliced), ¼ cup baby spinach, and 1 tablespoon crumbled feta cheese on 2 pieces Outer Aisle cauliflower sandwich thins
Dinner	1 (4-ounce) ribeye steak topped with 2 tablespoons crumbled blue cheese and 7 stalks roasted asparagus
Snack	1 serving Kite Hill almond milk yogurt with ¼ cup frozen wild blueberries
DAY 7	
Breakfast	Banana Walnut Overnight Oats (see recipe)
Lunch	½ cup cauliflower rice with 1 (4-ounce) cooked chicken breast and ½ cup steamed broccoli topped with Wildbrine Spicy Kimchi Sriracha
Dinner	⅓ cup ground turkey, ⅓ cup sweet potatoes, ¼ cup black beans, ¼ cup wild rice, and ½ cup kale sautéed in 1 tablespoon garlic butter
Snack	2 pickle spears wrapped in 2 nitrate-free deli turkey slices

VEGETARIAN MEAL PLAN

DAY 1	
Breakfast	2 eggs scrambled with ½ cup diced roasted sweet potatoes
Lunch	3 chopped hard-boiled eggs mixed with 1 tablespoon mayonnaise, and eaten with ½ medium zucchini (sliced)
Dinner	1 small baked potato topped with ½ cup black beans, ¼ cup salsa, ¼ medium avocado (chopped), and 1 tablespoon shredded Cheddar cheese
Snack	1 medium pink apple with 2 ounces sharp Cheddar cheese
DAY 2	
Breakfast	2 slices sprouted-grain toast with 2 tablespoons almond butter, ½ medium banana (sliced), and ⅛ teaspoon ground cinnamon
Lunch	½ cup cauliflower rice with ½ cup black beans and ½ cup steamed broccoli topped with Wildbrine Spicy Kimchi Sriracha
Dinner	½ cup cubed sweet potato, ½ cup black beans, ¼ cup wild rice, and ½ cup chopped kale sautéed in 1 tablespoon garlic butter
Snack	½ bell pepper sliced with 2 tablespoons spinach artichoke hummus
DAY 3	
Breakfast	¼ cup plain Greek yogurt topped with 1 tablespoon hempseeds, ¼ cup wild blueberries, 2 teaspoons peanut butter, and ⅛ teaspoon ground cinnamon
Lunch	2 cups mixed greens topped with ¼ cup kidney beans, ¼ medium avocado (sliced), 5 sliced strawberries, 1 tablespoon sliced almonds, 1 tablespoon crumbled feta cheese, and 2 tablespoons Tessemae's honey poppyseed dressing
Dinner	Stir-fry ½ cup tofu, 1 scrambled egg, ½ cup broccoli, ¼ cup diced red peppers, 2 tablespoons minced yellow onion, and ¼ cup cabbage and top with 2 tablespoons soy ginger sauce
Snack	½ cup cottage cheese with ¼ cup thawed frozen wild blueberries
DAY 4	
Breakfast	Pumpkin Walnut Overnight Oats (see recipe)
Lunch	2 slices gluten-free toast spread with 2 tablespoons hummus and topped with 6 raw cucumber slices, 4 tomato slices, ¼ cup chopped spinach, and ⅛ teaspoon lemon pepper

Dinner	1 cup chopped kale, 1 cup chopped spinach, ½ medium sliced apple, 1 tablespoon walnuts, 1 tablespoon crumbled feta cheese, and ⅓ cup kidney beans with 2 tablespoons vinaigrette dressing
Snack	1 Outer Aisle cauliflower sandwich thin topped with 1 tablespoon peanut butter
DAY 5	
Breakfast	2 slices sprouted-grain toast topped with ¼ medium avocado (mashed), sea salt, and black pepper
Lunch	1 cup chopped romaine lettuce topped with 2 chopped hard-boiled eggs mixed with 1 tablespoon mayonnaise, ¼ cup diced cucumber, 2 table-spoons diced tomato, and 1 tablespoon shredded Cheddar cheese
Dinner	1 medium baked sweet potato topped with ¼ cup pinto beans, ½ medium chopped avocado, chopped fresh cilantro, and 2 tablespoons tahini dressing
Snack	½ cup roasted pumpkin seeds
DAY 6	
Breakfast	Chocolate Strawberry Chia Pudding (see recipe)
Lunch	½ cup cooked quinoa mixed with ¼ cup chopped tomato, ¼ cup sliced roasted mushrooms, and ¼ cup roasted asparagus topped with 1 over-easy egg
Dinner	2 Outer Aisle cauliflower sandwich thins with ¼ cup pizza sauce, ¼ cup fresh mozzarella cheese chunks, fresh basil, and 4 tomato slices
Snack	½ cup plain unsweetened Greek yogurt with 1 tablespoon crushed wal-nuts and ¼ cup mixed berries
DAY 7	
Breakfast	Cinnamon Apple Quinoa Bowl (see recipe)
Lunch	1 large sprouted-grain tortilla with 2 tablespoons refried beans, ¼ cup salsa, ½ medium avocado (sliced), 1 tablespoon shredded Cheddar cheese, chopped fresh cilantro, and hot sauce
Dinner	2 cups mixed greens topped with 2 chopped hard-boiled eggs mixed with 1 tablespoon mayonnaise, ¼ medium avocado (diced), 2 tablespoons diced tomato, and 1 tablespoon shredded Cheddar cheese
Snack	2 cups air-popped popcorn sprinkled with 2 teaspoons nutritional yeast

VEGAN MEAL PLAN

DAY 1	
Breakfast	Mixed Berry Smoothie (see recipe)
Lunch	½ cup cooked polenta topped with ¼ cup roasted chickpeas, ½ cup sautéed sliced mushrooms and spinach, and drizzled with 2 teaspoons olive oil
Dinner	1 small baked potato topped with ½ cup black beans, ¼ cup salsa, ¼ medium avocado (chopped), and 1 tablespoon vegan queso
Snack	3 Medjool dates sliced open and stuffed with 2 tablespoons peanut butter

DAY 2	
Breakfast	Pumpkin Walnut Overnight Oats (see recipe)
Lunch	1 large sprouted-grain tortilla packed with ¼ cup chickpeas, ¼ cup kimchi, ¼ cup shredded carrots, ¼ cup chopped red pepper, and 2 teaspoons hoisin sauce
Dinner	½ cup cooked quinoa mixed with ¼ cup chopped tomato, ¼ cup sliced roasted mushrooms, and ¼ cup roasted asparagus
Snack	½ cup chopped thawed frozen mango topped with 1 teaspoon coconut cream

DAY 3	
Breakfast	2 slices sprouted-grain toast topped with 2 tablespoons almond butter and drizzled with 1 teaspoon honey
Lunch	2 cups chopped romaine lettuce topped with ¼ cup black beans, ¼ cup chopped bell peppers, ¼ cup grape tomatoes, ¼ medium avocado (chopped), 1 tablespoon sliced black olives, and 1 tablespoon crushed baked tortilla chips; add 2 tablespoons dressing of your choice
Dinner	Stir-fry ½ cup tofu, ½ cup broccoli, ¼ cup diced red pepper, 1 tablespoon chopped yellow onion, and ¼ cup shredded cabbage topped with 2 tablespoons soy ginger sauce
Snack	½ medium zucchini (sliced), served with 2 tablespoons garlic hummus

DAY 4	
Breakfast	Anti-Inflammatory Smoothie (see recipe)
Lunch	½ cup cooked brown rice mixed with ¼ cup black beans, ½ cup diced roasted sweet potato, and ½ cup chopped kale, topped with Wildbrine Spicy Kimchi Sriracha

Dinner	⅓ cup roasted chickpeas, ½ cup diced roasted sweet potato, 1 cup finely chopped kale, ¼ cup chopped cherry tomatoes, and 1 tablespoon minced red onion, topped with 2 tablespoons tahini sauce or green goddess dressing
Snack	1 medium banana (sliced) topped with 1 tablespoon melted coconut butter and 1 tablespoon unsweetened shredded coconut

DAY 5

Breakfast	½ cup cooked oatmeal topped with ½ large banana (sliced), ¼ cup crushed walnuts, 1 tablespoon maple syrup, and ⅛ teaspoon ground cinnamon
Lunch	2 cups chopped arugula topped with 1 tablespoon sliced almonds, ¼ cup sliced grapes, ½ cup roasted broccoli, ½ cup Italian-style tofu, and 2 tablespoons lemon vinaigrette dressing
Dinner	1 cup cooked lentil pasta topped with ½ cup sautéed spinach and ½ cup roasted garlic marinara sauce
Snack	½ cup roasted chickpeas

DAY 6

Breakfast	Tofu Scramble (see recipe)
Lunch	2 slices gluten-free toast spread with 2 tablespoons hummus and topped with ½ medium cucumber (sliced), ¼ cup diced tomato, ½ cup chopped fresh spinach, and ⅛ teaspoon lemon pepper
Dinner	1 medium baked sweet potato topped with ¼ cup pinto beans, ½ medium avocado (chopped), chopped fresh cilantro, and 2 tablespoons tahini dressing
Snack	¼ cup guacamole with ⅓ cup plantain chips

DAY 7

Breakfast	PB&J Overnight Oats (see recipe)
Lunch	1 large sprouted-grain tortilla with 2 tablespoons refried beans, ¼ cup salsa, ½ medium avocado (sliced), chopped fresh cilantro, and hot sauce
Dinner	1 cup cooked spaghetti squash topped with ¼ cup chickpeas, ½ cup sautéed spinach, and ¼ cup vegan Alfredo sauce or pesto sauce
Snack	1 medium apple (sliced) with 2 tablespoons almond butter

Resources

Diet Doctor

www.dietdoctor.com

This website is a great resource for information about intermittent fasting and low-carb/keto life-styles. There are short videos that answer commonly asked questions, as well as resources for different types of meal plans.

The Honest Guys

www.thehonestguys.co.uk

If you want to incorporate guided meditations into your stress-relief program, The Honest Guys offer videos of various lengths, from a few minutes to a couple of hours. Videos are tailored to everything from basic stress relief to addressing phobias.

Institute for Functional Medicine

www.ifm.org

If you think you have a hormonal problem that requires the intervention of a healthcare practitioner, you can use the "locate a practitioner" tool to find a functional medicine doctor or a functionally trained nutritionist near you. These practitioners can provide testing, order high-quality supplements, and/or guide you through the steps to reduce your stress levels and prepare your body for intermittent fasting.

PaleOMG

https://paleomg.com

This website is an excellent resource for clean, Paleo-style recipes. Most recipes are easy to make, with ingredients you probably already have in your kitchen. They're also easy to transform into other diet plans—for example, by swapping out beef for beans—so even if you're not Paleo, it's a great start for some clean eating ideas.

Pinterest
www.pinterest.com

This website is one of the best resources for new recipes and meal plans. Just type what you're looking for into the search bar— e.g., "low-carb chili recipe"—and you'll be directed to hundreds of websites and blogs with results that match your search. It's also a great place to find workout plans.

Pure Haven
https://purehaven.com/lindsayboyers

Here, you'll find a complete line of nontoxic home and beauty products. Everything is free of endocrine-disrupting chemicals, and most ingredients are organic.

WebMD Food Calculator
www.webmd.com/diet/
healthtool-food-calorie-counter

WedMD offers a free food calculator that shows the full nutrition facts for popular food items and dishes from popular restaurants and chains.

Yoga with Adriene
https://yogawithadriene.com

Yoga with Adriene is run by Adriene Mishler, an international yoga teacher from Austin, Texas. She posts free videos for yogis in all stages that you can access through her website and on *YouTube*. If you're new to yoga, or you've tried it before but couldn't get into it, give Adriene's content a try. You also have the option of joining a paid subscription service where you get access to premium features.

US/Metric Conversion Chart

VOLUME CONVERSIONS	
US Volume Measure	Metric Equivalent
⅛ teaspoon	0.5 milliliter
¼ teaspoon	1 milliliter
½ teaspoon	2 milliliters
1 teaspoon	5 milliliters
½ tablespoon	7 milliliters
1 tablespoon (3 teaspoons)	15 milliliters
2 tablespoons (1 fluid ounce)	30 milliliters
¼ cup (4 tablespoons)	60 milliliters
⅓ cup	90 milliliters
½ cup (4 fluid ounces)	125 milliliters
⅔ cup	160 milliliters
¾ cup (6 fluid ounces)	180 milliliters
1 cup (16 tablespoons)	250 milliliters
1 pint (2 cups)	500 milliliters
1 quart (4 cups)	1 liter (about)
WEIGHT CONVERSIONS	
US Weight Measure	Metric Equivalent
½ ounce	15 grams
1 ounce	30 grams
2 ounces	60 grams
3 ounces	85 grams
¼ pound (4 ounces)	115 grams
½ pound (8 ounces)	225 grams
¾ pound (12 ounces)	340 grams
1 pound (16 ounces)	454 grams

OVEN TEMPERATURE CONVERSIONS	
Degrees Fahrenheit	**Degrees Celsius**
200 degrees F	95 degrees C
250 degrees F	120 degrees C
275 degrees F	135 degrees C
300 degrees F	150 degrees C
325 degrees F	160 degrees C
350 degrees F	180 degrees C
375 degrees F	190 degrees C
400 degrees F	205 degrees C
425 degrees F	220 degrees C
450 degrees F	230 degrees C
BAKING PAN SIZES	
American	**Metric**
8 × 1½ inch round baking pan	20 × 4 cm cake tin
9 × 1½ inch round baking pan	23 × 3.5 cm cake tin
11 × 7 × 1½ inch baking pan	28 × 18 × 4 cm baking tin
13 × 9 × 2 inch baking pan	30 × 20 × 5 cm baking tin
2 quart rectangular baking dish	30 × 20 × 3 cm baking tin
15 × 10 × 2 inch baking pan	30 × 25 × 2 cm baking tin (Swiss roll tin)
9 inch pie plate	22 × 4 or 23 × 4 cm pie plate
7 or 8 inch springform pan	18 or 20 cm springform or loose bottom cake tin
9 × 5 × 3 inch loaf pan	23 × 13 × 7 cm or 2 lb narrow loaf or pate tin
1½ quart casserole	1.5 liter casserole
2 quart casserole	2 liter casserole

Index

About the Author

Lindsay Boyers, CHNC, is a holistic nutritionist specializing in the ketogenic diet, gut health, mood disorders, and functional nutrition. Lindsay earned a degree in food and nutrition from Framingham State University, and she holds a certificate in holistic nutrition consulting from the American College of Healthcare Sciences. She has written fifteen books and has had more than two thousand articles published across various websites, including *mindbodygreen*, *CNET*, *Forbes*, *Healthline*, *Livestrong*, *The Spruce Eats*, and *Verywell Health*, among others. Lindsay truly believes that you can transform your life through food, a proper mindset, and shared experiences, and that's what she aims to convey to her readers.